HAPPY BACK

Learn What Causes Neck and Back Pain, and How to Avoid Pain on Your Own

Dr. Scott Fuller, *DC, CCST, DACNB*

HAPPY BACK
Learn What Causes Neck and Back Pain,
and How to Avoid Pain on Your Own
by Dr. Scott Fuller

Published by:
Health Works Publishing
576 Main Street
Woburn, MA 01801 U.S.A.

Printed and bound in Canada.

Interior Photographs: Dr. Scott Fuller
Model: Ann Coros
Cover and Interior Design/Composition: Brian Moore
Cover and Interior Images: Brian Moore, Stefan Gandl/*Neubau Welt,*
and iStockphoto

Publisher's Cataloging-in-Publication
(Provided by Quality Books, Inc.)

Fuller, Scott, 1966-
Happy back : learn what causes neck and back pain,
and how to avoid pain on your own / Scott Fuller.
p. cm.
Includes bibliographical references and index.
LCCN 2007923514
ISBN-13: 978-0-9792608-0-3
ISBN-10: 0-9792608-0-9

1. Backache--Prevention. 2. Back--Care and hygiene.
3. Neck pain--Prevention. 4. Neck--Care and hygiene.
I. Title.

RD771.B217F85 2007   617.5′64
QBI07-600080

DEDICATION

This book is dedicated to those that have endured suffering, those that are searching for conservative solutions, and those interested in prevention.

PREFACE: HOW TO USE THIS BOOK

You are welcome to read this book cover to cover or you can flip around and read topics as you like. The table of contents will help you navigate ideas. The book is full of pictures which will hopefully help with explanations.

I welcome your feedback, so if you have suggestions for future publications, please see the contact information at the back of the book.

Chiropractors, physicians, physical therapists, acupuncturists, massage therapists, and individual purchasers may copy single pages or chapters for instructional use for patients, clients, and friends. Please do not reproduce the whole book for distribution.

ADDITIONAL LEARNING MATERIALS

CD's and DVD's of the information in Happy Back will be available, as well as updated editions of the book in the future. Please contact us if you are interested. Contact information is at the back of the book. You can provide us with your name, address, phone number and/or your e-mail address.

ACKNOWLEDGEMENTS

Several people helped make my ideas presentable to you.

Special thanks to Dr. Dan Murphy for his expertise, commitment, and research over the years. Thank you to many of my colleagues for their input and wisdom, including Dr. Don Harrison, Dr. Dwight DeGeorge, Dr. Robert Melillo, Dr. Dave Burgdorf, Dr. Peter Percuoco, Dr. Mark Alano, Dr. Phil Arnone, and Dr. Ted Carrick, among others.

I wish to express special gratitude to Terry Marotta, who is an incredible writer, speaker, and thinker, and who helped tirelessly edit this text. She also provided much needed motivation to complete my first work.

I am deeply indebted to Sally Edwards for her inspiration, ideas, and experience. She is also a gifted athlete and author.

Many others helped polish this text, and provided valuable input. Thanks to Doug Fuller his time and input, Scott B. and Marshall W. for their ideas and energy, Ann Coros for her generous time and skill, and Brian Moore for his design expertise and hard work.

Thank you to my mother for her never-ending support, patience, and enthusiasm.

Thank you to the Bally Total Fitness Club of Woburn, MA for use of their facility for gym photographs.

Additionally, thanks to all of my patients who inspired me to work harder and to be the best doctor of chiropractic I can be. They unknowingly urged me to find solutions and prevention measures for their difficulties, which ultimately led to this publication, and hopefully many more to come.

Yours in Health, Wellness, and Prevention,

Dr. Scott Fuller, D.C.

*"Part of my job
is to make
part of my job
go away."*

SCOTT FULLER, D.C.

TABLE OF CONTENTS

For more information and healthy advice, please visit Dr. Fuller's website:

www.drscottfuller.com

INTRODUCTION

This book is written out of both inspiration and frustration. I am inspired by the courage and valor of all people facing serious health issues. I am also inspired by the ability of the human body's complex machinery to repair and regenerate. I am a frustrated healthcare practitioner in that most of the problems for which people seek treatment are highly preventable. They are preventable with such activities and strategies as increased flexibility, better body mechanics and ergonomics, and maintenance/wellness visits to a chiropractor, which help prevent problems from returning.

When I first opened my own practice in 1993 I instructed each patient to do ten minutes of spinal specific exercises twice a day, morning and night. These exercises were designed to improve spinal flexibility, reduce the accumulation of day-to-day spinal stress, improve posture, maintain spinal wellness, and decrease pain and the chance of future problems. However, many patients did not follow through with these exercises. People are busy, and after the pain is gone, often the exercise program stops. In an effort to have more people follow through with exercises, I designed a program that only takes a few minutes a day, which I will share with you. As a result, my minimum recommendation decreased to just over one minute of spinal exercises both in the morning and evening (not including periodic exercises throughout the day, and ergonomic changes, which you will learn). In my opinion, this minimum exercise program can still provide the benefits you need and are searching for.

If the only thing you take away from this book is the few exercises that occupy only a little over a minute in the morning and evening, this book will be well worth your investment. The focus of this book is not chiropractic, although chiropractic is an important part of your healthcare. Rather, the focus is to teach you things you can do on your own to reduce the chances of having acute and chronic problems with your spine and to add years to your life as well as life to your years.

Spinal trauma occurs in everyday life but often goes unnoticed, without pain until later in life. Spinal trauma also begins early in life with birth trauma, even with births that are considered normal. Children fall when they learn to walk, and then they run, play and fall. Children and young adults sit at school desks with their heads down and shoulders rounded for hours each day, for 12-20 years.

Ongoing spinal stress and trauma occur with all sports and activities such as football, hockey, gymnastics, field hockey, softball, track, soccer, wrestling, intramural sports, baseball, cheerleading, band, and triathlons. As adults, most of us sit nearly motionless at desks and in front of computers with the same poor posture that took its toll when we were in school – that is, head down, shoulders rounded, accentuated hump in the middle back. If you have a physically demanding job, whether you are a full-time mom/dad or a land-scaper, trash collector or a construction worker, irritation and trauma to your spine and body are ongoing issues. Indulging in weekend warrior athletics and performing chores around your home add insult to injury. No wonder so many of us flood chiropractic, physical therapy, massage therapy and medical offices with neck and back pain.

It would serve humankind greatly if we could all learn techniques to re-duce, remove and counteract this spinal damage to reduce our pain, suffering and disability. I write this book for the purpose of decreasing and preventing needless suffering, and to save you time, pain, and money.

This book will provide you with useful methods to reduce irritation to your spine and nervous system and, ultimately, improve your health overall. Another goal I have is to help you reduce spinal arthritis and degeneration. Spinal arthritis is common, but not normal. Because spinal arthritis and pain are so common, they are *considered* normal and seen as an unavoidable con-sequence of aging. However, the amount and speed of spinal degeneration is something that is controllable. If deterioration and arthritis of the spine be-come significant enough, your work, relationships, sports and playtime will suffer. As with any human ailment, prevention is the key to a healthy spine and a healthy life. I will provide you with a plan of spinal care and mainte-nance you can begin upon immediately, which will hopefully lead to greater health and happiness for you and your family.

Both of my parents had "bad backs," and both sought out chiropractic care for relief. When I was in my early teens, my parents' chiropractor posed the thought: "Why leave your kids at home to suffer the same fate as you?" Thus the Fuller children began receiving chiropractic care at an earlier age than most, and I pass along the same thought to you. It is never too early (or too late) to engage in healthy, illness-prevention strategies. Although many people use chiropractic care as an emergency pain relief service, chiropractic's best benefit is to work toward preventing future problems, especially with the care of children. In my office, treatment of children focuses on proper spinal flexibility and biomechanics during growth and development, even if children do not have illnesses or complaints. Children begin to learn from me important exercise, ergonomic, and dietary habits that can stay with them for a lifetime.

This style of service falls under the category of true health care, being a program of promoting health and wellness, instead of trying to fix things that are broken. The analogies that can be used to illustrate this point are endless. We change the oil in our cars even though the cars are running fine, in an effort to minimize engine wear and tear and decrease the chance of a major breakdown. We see our dentist regularly before our teeth hurt, to try to prevent tooth and gum problems. It can be useful to adopt the philosophies of auto and tooth maintenance and apply them to the health of the spine and the entire body. After people feel well again, I continuously encourage follow-through of some flexibility and postural exercises and the ergonomic habits you will learn about in this book. I also suggest that people consider wellness and maintenance visits to a chiropractor in an effort to reduce the chances of having future problems. Unfortunately, many people do not return for care and often the same or similar problems return, especially if they stop doing their "homework" after they feel well again. Please consider following through with the simple strategies described in this book so you can have a Happy Back.

If you have neck, back, arm, or leg pain, your first question is probably "What's wrong with me?"

I will address this question first, and this is the first question I try to answer when patients come to my office.

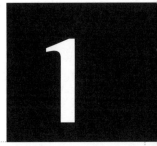

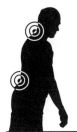

WHAT HURTS AND WHY?

TISSUES THAT CAUSE PAIN

I begin your first office visit with a thorough health history. Immediately after taking the history, I offer a tentative diagnosis and explain, in simple, unscientific terms, what I think is causing your problem. In the vast majority of low back and neck pain cases, irritation of the intervertebral discs and joints (to be detailed later) are the most common sources of pain. It is well documented in medical research that discs and joints, not muscles, are the common sources of acute and chronic pain in the neck and low back. The muscles, however, are involved in spinal dysfunction, therefore, muscle imbalances and scar tissue must also be addressed to achieve maximum improvements.

The muscles of your body have a rich blood supply. If they are injured, regeneration and repair is generally swift and the muscle injury itself is rarely a source of chronic pain. In contrast, discs are mostly *avascular* (no blood supply), and ligaments and joints by nature have a poor blood supply. The ability to bring oxygen and nutrients to discs and joints is poor; therefore repair is slow and often inadequate. Damage to the discs and joints from injuries, neglect, and abuse is repaired with scar tissue. Scar tissue is like a cheap grade of the original tissue; it is weaker, less flexible and more pain-sensitive than the original. After years of abuse from poor posture and ergonomics, sports, injuries and immobility, neck and back pain may become chronic. Muscles may *contribute* to spinal pain syndromes and disc and joint dysfunction, but muscles are rarely the primary source of pain. Many people erroneously believe, or are told, that their back and neck pain is caused from "pulled muscles."

"Doctor Fuller, I think I pulled a muscle in my back/neck," is a common statement from new patients. In simple terms, I give most of my neck, low back, arm and leg pain patients the diagnosis of "irritated discs and joints, with spinal subluxations." This simply and clearly states the *likely* sources of pain.

RADIATING PAIN

If you have neck and back pain, you may also have pain that radiates to other areas, which is also called *referred pain*. A neck problem may refer pain to the shoulders and arms, and a low back problem may refer pain to the buttocks and legs. An incorrect *"pinched nerve"* diagnosis is often times given as the reason for referred pain. In most cases of neck pain and low back pain with pain down the arms or legs, nerves are <u>not</u> being pinched. Actual pinched or *compressed nerves* are rare and generally have clearly identifiable signs. Muscle weakness and *atrophy*, loss of *vibration sensation*, loss of *reflexes* and loss of *pain and temperature sensations* along the involved nerve pathway are clues that nerve compression may be occurring. Nerve compression, or a pinched nerve, can be caused by a variety of mechanisms, but in the spine it is most commonly caused by a *herniated disc* or *bone spur* actually pressing on a nerve root. Some of these cases do require surgical decompression, but because pinched nerves are so rare as compared to other causes of pain, the discussion here will focus on the common causes of spine and referred pain, which are mostly avoidable. These strategies can also help prevent nerve compression from occurring in the first place by reducing the chances of herniated discs, osteoarthritis, and bone spur formation.

Nerves can also become compressed in other locations in the arms and legs. For example, *Median nerve* compression at the wrist is called *carpal tunnel syndrome*. Many of these types of compressions, sometimes called *peripheral nerve entrapments* respond well to chiropractic care and other conservative treatments such as physical therapy and massage therapy.

HOW DOES THE DAMAGE OCCUR?

In my office I regularly hold a "health class" specifically designed for new patients, or people with questions about chiropractic and health in general.

This 45-60 minute program is full of useful information similar to what you read here. One important subject I always cover is how discs, joints, and muscles become damaged and painful. The activities of everyday life cause minor trauma (*microtrauma*) and irritation to our spinal tissues, and these accumulate over time. Sports activities, lifting, sitting, driving, and cleaning the house, especially when performed with poor posture, are sources of ongoing spinal damage. As we are in the computer age, the head down, shoulders-rounded, immobile positions we assume in front of computers compounds the situation. Childhood traumas and injuries, and even the birth process itself, are additional factors that damage the spine. The accumulation of these irritants and injuries takes a toll on the healthy condition of discs and joints. In addition, many of us are not physically active and the typical American diet, loaded with bad fat, too much protein, processed food, and additives, adds extra weight, which causes additional joint and tissue insult. This typical American diet also promotes inflammation, leading to more pain and arthritis. As I discuss in Chapter 16 (Arthritis), animal protein is an additional tissue and joint irritant. Smokers suffer from more wear and tear arthritis, and smokers tend to heal at a slower rate than non-smokers. All of these factors are the recipe for spinal breakdown and chronic pain.

HEALING THE DAMAGE

The body mends damaged discs, joints, and muscles via a three-step process[1,2]. After an injury, the *acute inflammation stage* occurs, which lasts approximately three days. Damaged tissues bleed and swell, and become hot, red and painful. The *repair/regeneration stage* follows during which new tissue is produced. This new scar tissue is weaker, stiffer, and more sensitive to pain than the original. The third step in the healing process is the *remodeling stage* where tissue fibers become oriented along the lines of stress and strain in an effort to reorganize more closely to the original. This healing response occurs as a result of a singular traumatic event, or from continuous microtrauma. The more scar tissue, the more weakness, stiffness, and pain. Many tend to blame these chronic problems on old age. However, I have seen clearly observable disc damage on X-rays of people in their twenties. At the same time, I have also observed a lack of arthritic joints in people many decades older. These observations should suggest to us that (all types of) arthritis is not a function of age. Rather, the challenge is to reduce trauma (macro and micro), restore individual joint and disc function through motion, improve posture, increase flexibility, and reduce dietary consumption of *saturated, hydrogenated, and trans-fats,* animal protein and processed food. Appropriate *motion therapy* is essential for post-trauma healing and to relieve chronic postural stress. Many of us lose spinal flexibility throughout our lives and this stiffening allows more of the inflammation/repair/remodeling processes to occur, resulting in more scar tissue, dysfunction and pain.

CONSIDER CHIROPRACTIC

Dr. Dan Murphy is one of the most notable, respected doctors in the chiropractic profession, and is an accomplished lecturer and author. His explanation of chiropractic is one of the best: "A chiropractor offers something unique and special to humankind, which is called an adjustment. The chiropractic spinal adjustment stretches injured and scarred areas fully, where active and passive motion and stretching cannot. Also, individual joint and disc problems may not be corrected by exercise and stretching alone. Unfortunately, it is known that stretching and exercising across a joint that is dysfunctional may actually lead to accelerated deterioration."[3]

I explain it to people this way: Chiropractic adjustments stimulate the powerful nerve network within spinal tissues. These adjustments stimulate the numerous specialized nerve endings called *receptors* in spinal joints, discs and other tissues. Although I will not discuss detailed science, it is important to know some basics. These nerve receptors, called *mechanoreceptors and muscle spindles* are stimulated by joint and muscle motion and gravity. If all the discs, joints and muscles of the spine are healthy and moving properly, these receptors will flood the nervous system with important and healthy nerve traffic. If joints, discs and muscles of the spine are stiff and immobile, the amount of receptor traffic to the nervous system is decreased and may adversely affect the health of the nervous system. When this motion traffic is reduced, it may be replaced with pain. Chiropractic adjustments, along with appropriate flexibility exercises, ergonomics, posture control, and other therapies, are focused on joint health. Improved joint and muscle health will help restore appropriate receptor stimulation of the nervous system for improved overall health, function, and decreased pain.

REVIEW

Irritated discs and joint tissues cause the vast majority of neck and back pain. These tissues become irritated and injured from everyday activities and events such as childhood and childbirth traumas, sports, poor posture, prolonged sitting, improper lifting and cleaning, and exercising improperly. The accumulation of trauma, stress, and injury leads to scar tissue formation, stuck and "glued" joints and, ultimately, pain. The keys to treating and preventing these problems are increased flexibility, exercise, chiropractic adjustments, rehabilitation, improved posture, and ergonomic habits. This book will help provide you with some of these keys. These strategies also reduce the chances of chronic pain, disability, and suffering in the future so you can enjoy your work, relationships, sports, and playtime.

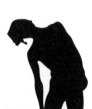

SPINAL FLEXIBILITY EXERCISES

"Danny" (not his real name), age 54, came to my office with an all-too-typical low back pain case, after lifting heavy items a year earlier. He waited to seek treatment, hoping the pain would go away, but the pain continued and returned frequently with minor activity. Chiropractic adjustments helped relieve his pain, but his back would still "go out" from time to time. He decided on his own to increase exercises 1, 2, and 4 (which you are about to learn) from the minimum recommended 10 reps, up to 100 reps each. After doing the exercises regularly for a month, he remarked how great his back felt. He has since reduced the reps to about 50 each, and in combination with wellness chiropractic treatments, his back has been considerably better.

One key to a healthy spine is flexibility. In my office I teach and encourage daily spinal motion exercises. When I first started practicing chiropractic I taught exercises that took ten minutes in the morning and ten minutes at night. Through my experience I found out that most people were not following through with these exercises, so I reduced the exercise time to about one minute. I consider this recommendation a bare minimum and actually encourage you to do much more. I advise you to consult with your doctor before beginning these exercises. These exercises are not <u>replacements</u> for chiropractic adjustments. They work best along <u>with</u> chiropractic adjustments.

Each exercise should be performed at a comfortable pace and intensity. I recommend these four exercises be done first thing in the morning when you wake up. This will form a habit and ensure that these exercises are performed daily. You may be stiffer in the morning, so use care not to push these exercises too far. Exercising and stretching first thing in the morning will help wake you up and prepare your spine for the day ahead. Some of you prefer to do the exercises later in the morning after a warm shower, and this is fine as long as you create the habit of doing the exercises daily. Remember that each exercise should be performed in a comfortable, pain-free zone. If you feel pain during any exercise, you've gone too far. Reduce the amount of motion and try again. If the exercise continues to cause pain, stop the exercise immediately. People who have acute, sharp, or intense pain <u>should not perform these exercises and should be evaluated immediately by a doctor.</u>

There are many other exercises you can do that are beneficial. Some of you have been to therapists and chiropractors and have been taught a variety of exercises, but in my experience most people do not follow through after the pain is gone. Home rehabilitation programs are often too time consuming or difficult, resulting in many home programs being abandoned, especially after the pain is gone. I want to get you started with a few excellent but brief exercises that you can do daily to help you achieve a healthier, pain-free spine.

<u>Exercise 1: The Spinal Twist</u> (Figures 2-1 through 2-3)

Intervertebral discs love rotation. Their criss-crossed fiber pattern (drawing 1)[4] responds well to rotational motion. This exercise is best performed in the sitting position, but can be done standing as well. Spread your feet apart, feet on the floor, sit up straight with your shoulders back and your chin a little higher than usual. Place your arms out in front of you at shoulder level, if possible (Fig. 2-1). If you have a shoulder problem, you can lower your arms down to

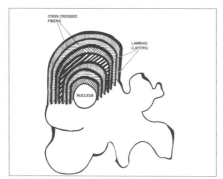

Drawing 1: Discs: Criss-Crossed Fibers

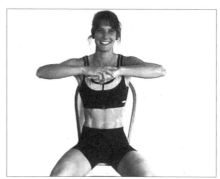

Fig. 2-1   Spinal twist - start

a comfortable level and even keep your hands on your hips, if necessary. You can leave your hands apart or clasp them together. Turn your body and head fully and comfortably to the right as if you are looking over your right shoulder (Fig. 2-2), and then turn fully to the left without stopping in the middle (Fig. 2-3). Focus the twisting motion with the neck and lower spine, not your arms. Do not perform the twist too quickly as you could hurt yourself. Twist at a comfortable pace and turn to the left and to the right ten times each way. Do one set of spinal twists in the morning and one at night. If you have a long commute and a sit-down job, you may find doing these twists twice per day is inadequate. You may benefit from doing a set when you arrive at work and occasionally during the day to counteract the lack of motion of prolonged sitting, both of which increase disc and joint irritation. Please start these exercises slowly and increase the amount of exercise per day as you feel better and gain flexibility. Doing too much too quickly can be detrimental.

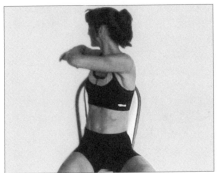

Fig. 2-2   Spinal twist - right   *Fig. 2-3   Spinal twist - left*

Exercise 2: The Side Bend (Figures 2-4 through 2-6)

This exercise is best performed in a sitting position, but can be done standing. Sit up straight, feet far apart, shoulders back and chin higher than normal with your hands resting on your thighs (Fig. 2-4). Bend as far as comfortably possible to the right, also gently bending your head to the right as if you were bringing your right ear to your right shoulder (Fig. 2-5). Once again, keep this exercise in the comfortable zone. If it hurts, you have gone too far so back off. Next, bend as far as comfortably possible to the left, also bending the neck to the left (Fig. 2-6), without stopping in the middle. Perform this side bend exercise ten times to each side, moving in a constant flowing motion. After doing a set, if you wish you can also bend to each side and hold that stretch for a period of time, for 5-10 seconds. Begin with one set in the morning and one set at night. This is the absolute minimum recommendation. Increase the frequency of the exercise during the day as it becomes comfortable and your flexibility improves, and to break up the accumulation of spinal stress with prolonged sitting.

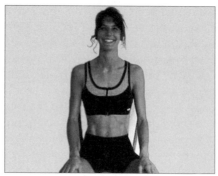

Fig. 2-4   Side bend - start

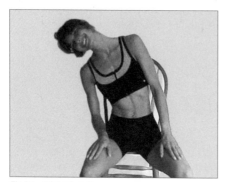

Fig. 2-5   Side bend - right

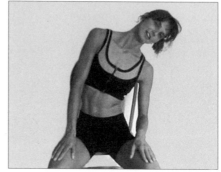

Fig. 2-6   Side Bend - left

Exercise 3: Spinal Extension (Figures 2-7 through 2-10)

This is a posture improvement exercise. Most of you should place significant importance on this exercise as it will help reduce and prevent the slouching posture that is all too common and quite preventable. Some doctors and therapists have reservations about this exercise, but there is no need to fear bending your head back. The biomechanical and neurological research supporting the goal of this exercise is extensive. Logically, if almost all people slump forward as they get older (Fig. 2-7), performing activities in the opposite direction in an effort to prevent or reduce this slouching makes sense. Remember, when looking at the neck (*cervical spine*) from the side (Fig. 2-8)[5], it is supposed to have a forward curve, which allows for an easy ability to bend the head back.

This exercise is best performed sitting, but if you have good balance it can be done standing as well. Place your hands behind you in your lower back area with your elbows almost straight (Fig. 2-9). Clasp one hand with the other. Slowly and carefully pull your shoulders directly backwards as far as you comfortably can, as if you are trying to pinch something between your shoulder blades. Lift your chin back as far as you comfortably can without pain (Fig. 2-10). If this hurts your neck, shoulder, or other areas, you have gone too far so back off. Hold this extension position for ten seconds. Do two or more of these in the morning and two or more at night. If you sit most of the day, especially looking at computers, do this exercise frequently throughout the day. Slowly but steadily increase the frequency and intensity of this exercise during the day. Many of you with neck and shoulder complaints and stiffness will have to start slowly and pay close attention to performing the exercise within your comfort zone. Many of my patients who stick with this exercise notice improvements with posture and flexibility, and a decrease in pain and stiffness.

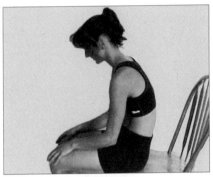

Fig. 2-7 *Slumpy - avoid!*

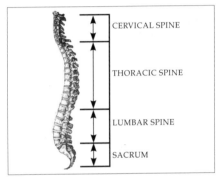

CERVICAL SPINE

THORACIC SPINE

LUMBAR SPINE

SACRUM

Fig. 2-8

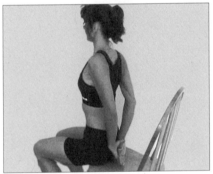

Fig. 2-9 *Spinal extension - Step 1*

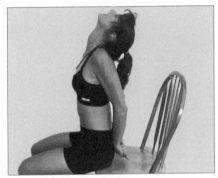

Fig. 2-10 *Spinal extension - Step 2*

Many of us work at a desk, sit at school desks, or at a computer. All of these positions promote a slumped-forward, head-forward, chin-down posture (Fig. 2-7). Over time the sitting posture wears down the discs, joints, muscles, and other tissues of the spine. Small wonder most of us feel pain, stiffness, and discomfort at the end of the day, and as we age. This exercise is designed to help minimize these problems. Due to our lifestyles and postures of having our head forward, we lose and often reverse the natural curve in our necks, making this extension more and more difficult to do. Many of us have trouble with this exercise in the beginning. As flexibility and structure improve the exercise will become easier and even enjoyable. Many of my patients have said that at first the exercise was uncomfortable, but as they continued, the exercise felt great to do! As with any exercise, start slow, be patient, and do it daily. The benefits are greater than I can describe here. Not only will your posture improve, but your ribcage will function better with the improved posture, making breathing and oxygen intake more efficient. Also, this improved posture and structure may decrease the occurrence and the effects of *osteoarthritis* (joint wear and tear).

The first three exercises described here can be effectively performed in the standing position (Figures 2-11 through 2-13). Please use extra caution when doing these exercises standing. Spread your feet apart for balance, and make sure there is adequate space around you, so you do not bang into objects or people. You may want to only twist at the waist and keep the head still when doing the spinal twist exercise standing, to maintain balance.

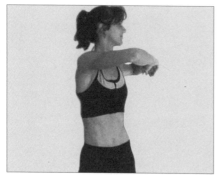

Fig. 2-11   *Standing spinal twist*

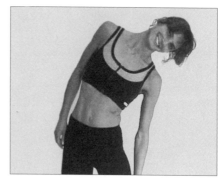

Fig. 2-12   *Standing side bend*

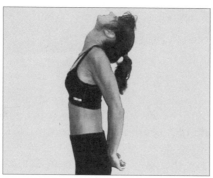

Fig. 2-13   *Standing spinal extension*

Exercise 4: Knee Roll (Figures 2-14 through 2-16)

I believe this is one of the best overall exercises one can do for improving the health of the discs and joints of the lower back. This exercise should be performed lying on your back on the floor. Doing it in bed is OK, but the floor is better. Most people perform this exercise at home or at the gym although a few of my patients have been known to find an empty conference room during the day to do some. Place your arms where you want, though out to the side for stability is probably best, and bend your knees, keeping your feet flat (Fig. 2-14). Roll both knees together to the right as far as comfortably possible (Fig. 2-15). Some of you will rotate your knees completely to the floor. Others will not be able to go as far, due to pain or stiffness. Then, rotate your knees to the left in a smooth motion, not too fast or slow (Fig. 2-16), and do not stop in the middle. As I mentioned before, you should perform this exercise in your comfortable zone only. Do not over-rotate and do not force the movement. If you hear joint noises (cracking sounds) during this or any of the other exercises, it is a normal consequence of exercising your joints through their full range of motion. Don't let the sound alarm you as it is perfectly normal. The sound is gas (CO_2) rushing between two joint surfaces as you gently stretch them apart, and the stretch is typically therapeutic for joint health, as long as the stretch

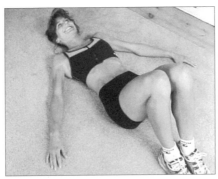

Fig. 2-14   Knee roll - start

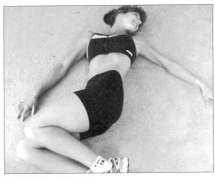

Fig. 2-15   Knee roll - right

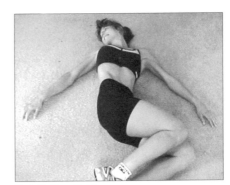

Fig. 2-16   Knee roll - left

and pop do not hurt. If you prefer, you can keep your head and neck still during the knee roll exercise.

As an important reminder these exercises should be performed under the supervision of your chiropractor, medical physician, or therapist. They are quite safe for almost everyone if performed as described here. All of them are focused on improving flexibility, and the spinal extension exercise is focused on improving structure and posture. There are hundreds of excellent exercises you could do that are beneficial, and you might have been taught exercises by your healthcare practitioner. It has been my experience that most people do not follow through with multiple exercises, but I believe many more people will follow through with just a few exercises each day. If you are already performing a program of stretching and strengthening exercises with a therapist or on your own, these exercises can be added to your program without interference. If you have an aversion to the word "exercise," then consider calling these stretches "healthy spinal procedures." You already exercise your teeth three times a day, so "brushing your spine" two or three times a day is reasonable. Remember, doing them first thing in the morning and just before you go to bed creates a new habit, which promotes regular follow-through of these exercises. Later in this book you will find additional exercises and healthy spinal procedures if you want to do more.

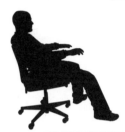

3

SITTING ERGONOMICS

Imagine looking at someone from the side, sitting in front of a computer. What do you see? You probably picture someone with their shoulders rounded, slouched forward, and their head jutting out towards the computer screen. Looks painful, doesn't it? When it comes to sitting in front of your computer all day, you know:

"ONE SIZE DOES NOT FIT ALL"

In discussing computer workstations with my brother Doug, he came up with this comment that "one size does not fit all" when it comes to ergonomics. When I talk about "ergonomics," I am referring to your body position and how you use your body and muscles during all of the tasks you perform during the day. He and I have discussed the ergonomics of his computer desk at work, which he has specifically designed for his body and posture. Being 6′ 4″ tall, he will have different needs than someone who is 5′ 2″. After he modified his workstation, personnel trained in ergonomics reviewed the changes. These people did not agree with the changes that he had made because they did not "fit" their ergonomic standards. That is when Doug reminded me that one size does not fit all, and that popular standards may not be appropriate for everybody. Keep in mind that you will want to work with my recommendations and make changes that are most comfortable for you. The recommendations I make about ergonomics are guidelines to begin making changes for both your spine and health. Please be flexible and make changes as you see fit. Also, keep in mind that what may feel comfortable to you now, due to your familiarity with it, may not be a good ergonomic position. A good example is the semi-reclined position many people use while driving. Poor car seat design and poor posture habits foster the slouched driving position. Although you may be comfortable with that position because it is so familiar, it is incorrect and contributes to spinal damage.

Much spinal injury and trauma is a result of cumulative degeneration due to poor posture, immobility, and how we use our bodies during our daily activities. Improving posture and ergonomics can reduce tremendous stress on your spinal discs, joints, and muscles. Discs and other spinal tissues thrive on motion. Prolonged sitting increases pressure on discs and decreases motion, which results in increased disc, joint, and muscle wear and eventually pain. Most of you have already figured out that the longer you sit, the more uncomfortable you become in your neck, upper back, and lower back. There are two main reasons for increased disc and joint irritation when you sit:

1. There is an increase in pressure on your discs when you sit. When you are lying down, there is about 15-17 pounds per square inch (psi) of pressure on your lumbar discs[6,7]. This is why many people with acute disc problems tend to feel somewhat better when lying down. When you are sitting or standing relaxed, there is 4-5 times as much pressure on your discs as compared to lying down. Bending forward while sitting or standing increases disc pressure by 8-10 times that of lying, and if you are lifting something when bent forward, the pressure increases considerably more.

2. When you are sitting, the discs, joints, and muscles are immobile. This lack of motion glues up the joints, wears down the discs, and does not stimulate motion nerve endings (called mechanoreceptors and muscle spindles), decreasing nerve traffic and power to the brain. Discs do not have a blood supply; they rely on transferring nutrients and waste products via osmosis. Osmosis is the absorption of materials from surrounding fluids, and osmotic activity depends on frequent motion all day long. Prolonged sitting decreases the ability of discs to absorb fluid and nutrients and eliminate wastes.

Many of us have jobs where we have to sit for prolonged periods. Because we cannot avoid all sitting, we need to employ a different strategy to reduce disc trauma and degeneration. I have several ideas you can use to reduce disc irritation and pain due to prolonged sitting:

1. **Frequent breaks** – Taking a frequent break is the most beneficial thing you can do to decrease disc stress. Standing up, even for a brief moment, can really help decrease the stress on your spine caused by sitting. Taking longer breaks with some walking is even better. If your workday requires eight hours sitting at a desk, I suggest getting out of your chair every 15 minutes, even if it is just for 5-10 seconds. You will feel significantly better throughout the day and you may even end up being more productive. Consider standing in meetings and conferences when possible. One of my patients with back pain has a sit-down job as a computer programmer. He used to take one break per hour and would walk around for a couple of minutes. My suggestion was for more frequent, shorter-duration breaks, which worked much better for him. Instead of one, two-minute break per hour, he now takes four, 30-second breaks every 15 minutes.

2. **Exercises** – Consider doing the exercises described in Chapter 2 frequently throughout the day. While sitting in your chair (or standing) you can take a 20-second break every 15 minutes and perform five spinal twists, five side bends, and one spinal extension. If you dare, you can even lie on the floor and do five knee rolls! I recommend doing one spinal extension exercise every 15 minutes (see Chapter 2, and don't forget to hold the extension position for ten seconds). This spinal extension exercise, if done regularly, will help relieve neck, shoulder and middle back stress, and keep your posture from slouching as you age.

CAR TRIPS

Long car trips require frequent breaks. I recommend a 3-5 minute break every hour to reduce disc and joint irritation. I realize that when you are taking a car trip, you want to press on to get to your destination faster. But wouldn't it be better to arrive at your destination five or ten or fifteen minutes later feeling comfortable and energetic rather than stiff, tight, sore and grumpy? I think these breaks are worth it. Plan ahead and leave a bit earlier so you can take them. At each stop I recommend a brisk walk for one or two minutes and a few of the twists, bends and extensions, which can be done standing. Consider taking breaks <u>before</u> you feel uncomfortable.

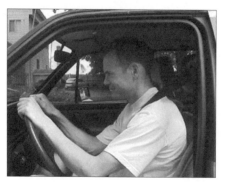

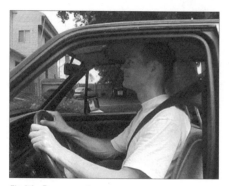

Fig. 3-1   Poor car posture   Fig. 3-2   Proper car posture

CAR SEAT POSITION

Please use care when setting the position of your car seat. You can contribute to poor posture and pain with poor car seat position (Fig. 3-1), or you can enhance proper posture and avoid a humpback with good car seat position (Fig. 3-2). Your headrest should be in the highest position it can be, and it should touch the back of your head as you drive to reduce neck injury if you are ever rear-ended. To promote good car posture, sit in your car first thing in the morning, nice and tall, and set your rearview mirror. This mirror position will encourage you to sit up straight each time you are in your car. The back of your seat should be as straight and upright as possible to promote proper posture and for additional protection. Also, if you have an airbag and if it were to ever deploy, you would want your body fully against your seat to minimize injury. If you are short and have short arms and legs, consider being as far away from the wheel as comfortably possible, again, to minimize the impact of the airbag.

PLANE TRIPS, SEMINARS

On plane trips you might consider an aisle seat so you can get up frequently for standing and stretching breaks. You can perform the side bend and twist-ing exercises when standing, and the spinal extension exercise when sitting. I frequently teach flight attendants and other passengers the simple stretches when they see me doing them. When I attend post-graduate classes and semi-nars, I sit near the back of the room so I can stand and stretch as frequently as I want without disturbing others. Try the exercises in the following section frequently when flying and sitting for long periods.

Sitting Aerobics (Figures 3-3 through 3-15)

There are other ways to increase flexibility and motion while sitting. I call this strategy "sitting aerobics." We naturally tend to squirm when sitting for a long time, as we do at the movies. I recommend performing sitting aerobics well <u>before</u> you get uncomfortable and fidgety. You can stretch your lower spine front and back by first pushing your chest and stomach out while pulling on your knees (Fig. 3-3) followed by pushing your lower back into the seat (Fig. 3-4). When you push your lower back into the seat, squeeze your abdominal muscles at the same time and this will increase the efficiency of this movement. Another stretch you can do is a side-to-side stretch. You can shift your body weight from the left to the right, back and forth (Figures 3-5 and 3-6). Pushing the right foot into the floor, squeezing your right thigh muscles and lifting the right side of your pelvis slightly off your seat can increase the efficiency of this movement. To rock in the other direction, push your left foot into the floor, contract your left thigh muscles, and lift the left side of the pelvis off the seat. You may notice you can stretch one side more easily than the other, so you may want to concentrate additional stretching on the difficult side.

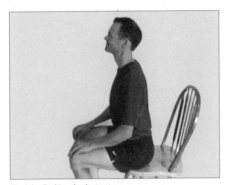

Fig. 3-3   *Pushing the chest out*

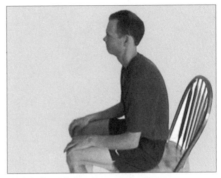

Fig. 3-4   *Stretch backwards*

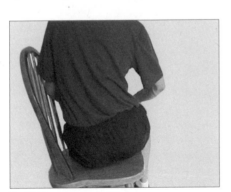

Fig. 3-5   *Lower back stretch - left*

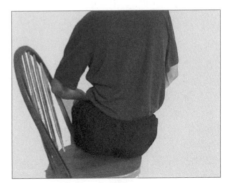

Fig. 3-6   *Lower back stretch - right*

Another helpful sitting maneuver to try is to move your pelvis in a circular motion as if you are using a hula-hoop. Rotate your pelvis this way in one direction a few times, and then reverse to the other direction. This motion can be augmented by moving your pelvis in a figure-eight motion, which is even more intricate than a circular motion. All of these activities can counteract much of the stiffness and stress that accumulate in the discs, joints and muscles of your spine while sitting.

The sitting position with the head down and shoulders rounded also places significant stress on the neck and middle back discs, joints and muscles. Years of sitting in school in this position followed by years of working at a desk and in front of a computer, accelerate degeneration in these areas. Frequent breaks to perform the spinal extension exercise described in Chapter 2 will help counteract stresses, and may help prevent some pain and joint wear in the neck, shoulders and middle back, and reduce the occurrence of headaches. If you have persistent neck problems, or are looking for additional stretches for the neck, you can perform the twisting and side-bending exercises isolating your head and neck, and increase their frequency each day (Figures 3-7 through 3-10).

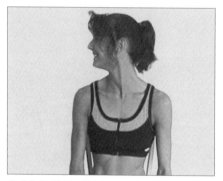

Fig. 3-7   Next twist - right

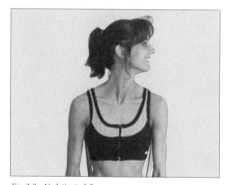

Fig. 3-8   Neck tiwst - left

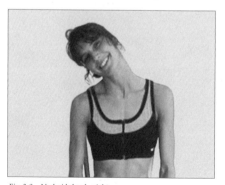

Fig. 3-9   Neck side bend - right

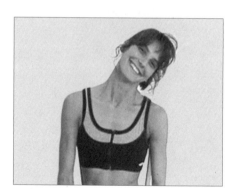

Fig. 3-10   Neck side bend - left

Please pay attention to the ergonomics of your work or school station. Computer monitors tend to be too low and should be placed slightly <u>above</u> eye level to promote slight extension of the head and neck (Fig. 3-11), which will help counteract the chin-down posture as you look at your keyboard, paperwork, and telephone. This new higher position is contrary to what most of you are used to, and will feel odd for a period of time as you adjust to it. Monitors placed at eye level are not high enough to provide this benefit, and most people seem to use them below eye level. Whenever possibly, try raising paperwork off the desk surface whenever possible. Try using an angled, drafting-style board to elevate paperwork to a higher position. For example, as I was working on this manuscript, I taped sheets of information I was reading from to a shelf above my head. Many computer devices, some of them attached to the monitor, help elevate material which reduces spinal stress and pain. When reading, try to hold items at eye level (Fig. 3-12), rather than having them low and flat (Fig. 3-13). If some items are too heavy to hold, such as textbooks, they can be propped up at an angle by leaning them on other books or a pillow (Fig. 3-14). Changing the organization of your workstation every month or two can help minimize daily stresses on your body. Mix up the placement of items at your desk such as the telephone, writing surface, keyboard, mouse, monitor, calculator, etc. If you do not utilize strategies like these, you may suffer the long-term adverse effects of stationary positions, including spinal arthritis, degenerating slumped posture, and chronic pain.

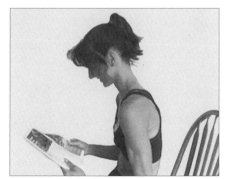

Fig. 3-11   Try raising your computer monitor

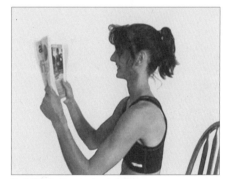

Fig. 3-12   Reading - good posture

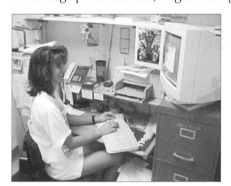

Fig. 3-13   Reading - bad posture

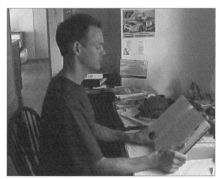

Fig. 3-14   Angle heavy books

If you sit for extended periods at a computer, you should consider making a standing work area in addition to the sitting workstation. Although it may be simple to construct, a standing workstation may not be possible for you. The only items that probably need to be repositioned are the keyboard and mouse, and many are now wireless. You might only need a small work surface above the desktop to raise the keyboard and mouse to allow you to work while standing. Being able to raise the monitor to eye level or above would also be helpful. When standing for long periods, the "spread eagle" position (to be described in the next chapter) will help eliminate additional stress.

Please be patient as you make these changes. It may take some time for you to unlearn the head-forward, chin-down position. Of course you cannot get totally away from having your chin down! For instance, when walking, you need to look down to see where you are going, but even this habit can change. (There is more on walking and running in Chapter 9.) You can decrease much of the daily spinal stress by becoming aware of the chin-down, head-forward posture with many of your daily activities. Minor changes in positions, coupled with the spinal exercises, can go a long way to reducing spinal wear and tear, arthritis and pain.

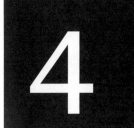

STANDING ISSUES

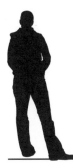

You are at a convention or a family gathering, standing around for hours. As the event continues, you notice your back begins to ache, and the ache gets worse and worse. You can't wait to sit down for some relief. Sound familiar? What is happening?

Standing motionless for extended periods of time can accumulate stress on the spine and associated soft tissues, accelerating disc and joint wear (degeneration and arthritis), which lead to pain. For example, a cook I saw as a patient injured his lower back discs, joints and muscles in an automobile accident. He missed some work due to the injury and pain, but luckily his injuries were minor and he was able to return to work shortly after he began seeing me for treatment. He came to my office the morning after he returned to work and said he had severe low back pain after standing in work for only one hour and suffered for the rest of the shift. I taught him a simple way to remove a lot of stress and pain while standing. I call this the "spread-eagle" position (Fig. 4-1). In contrast, standing with the feet close together and bending at the waist places adverse pressure on the lower back discs and joints (Fig. 4-2). If you spread the feet wide apart, as wide as comfortably possible, this decreases the forward lean at the waist needed to get you closer to your work surface. The next time this cook went back to work he tried this position and reported to me the next day that he had worked eight hours and had no increase in pain at all. It was so successful for him, he taught the other cooks this posture and all benefited!

Anyone can use this recommendation to decrease spinal stress during standing activities. At home when you are at your counter preparing food, washing dishes, cleaning or ironing (Fig. 4-3), utilize this spread-eagle position. People with other kinds of standing jobs will benefit greatly from this position as well. I understand that this position may seem a little unusual, but consider the benefits you gain with decreased spinal stress and reduced pain. The powerful thigh and gluteal muscles handle the pressure, as opposed to the low back muscles, and give you strength and endurance while in this position. As a reminder, when you feel pain in the standing position, it is not just the muscles that are the source of pain. The weight of the upper body leaning forward, coupled with the back muscles contracting in the back and pulling downward, lead to increased pressure on discs and joints, causing pain. By using the spread-eagle posture, the head forward and chin down posture is also minimized.

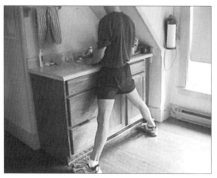
Fig. 4-1   "Spead-eagle" position - try it!

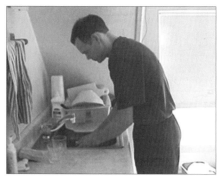
Fig. 4-2   Standing - poor posture

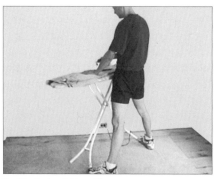
Fig. 4-3   Ironing - better position

If possible, try to raise your work surface. By placing materials higher up, you do not have to lean forward as much. This will not work in all situations, and it is impractical for most of us to remodel all of our home countertops. The spread-eagle posture will work wonders for you by reducing pressure and pain in situations when your work surface cannot be raised.

There are other situations where you may stand for long periods of time, for example shopping or standing in line, milling about at family gatherings and at conventions. The typical standing position with the knees locked and the pelvis tilted forward increases the low back (*lumbar*) curve (Fig. 4-4), increasing pressure on the posterior portion of the lower back discs and joints, causing pain for many of us. I fall into this category, and I get low back pain when standing in one place for a period of time. Some people have a decreased lower

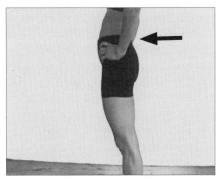

Fig. 4-4 *Too much low back curve*

back curve, and for them standing in this position is actually more comfortable. Wearing high heels accentuates the forward tilt and increases the curve even more. In my experience, some women are more comfortable with high heels, though this is the exception and not the rule, and is usually the case with women that have a loss of the lumbar curve (best evaluated with a standing lower back x-ray at a chiropractor's office). High heels will increase the lumbar curve to a more normal position in these cases, thus decreasing pain. Except for these rare cases, I recommend avoiding high heels whenever possible because of the additional lower back stress they cause for most women. Also, typical high-heeled shoes cause many serious foot problems, as many of these shoes are not shaped like the human foot. Unfortunately my mother has severe chronic daily foot pain, caused in large part by wearing pointed shoes for many years. She is now suffering, and would not have worn those shoes if she had known of the consequences.

I recommend changing the standing posture in a couple of ways. Bend the knees just slightly from full extension (Fig. 4-5). Also utilize a "pelvic tilt". Tuck your rear end down towards the floor and lift the front part of your pelvis up slightly by squeezing and contracting your ab muscles gently (Fig. 4-6). Both of these recommendations, bending the knees slightly and using the pelvic tilt, will decrease the lumbar curve and reduce the disc, joint, and muscle stress when standing. You can bend the knees and do a pelvic tilt subtly, without others noticing what you are doing.

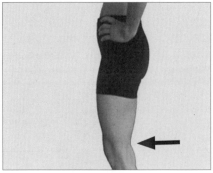

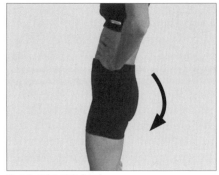

Fig. 4-5 *Bend the knees slightly*

Fig. 4-6 *Pelvic tilt backward*

An additional strategy to reduce back pain while standing is to place one foot on something that is elevated (Fig. 4-7). Put one foot up on a raised surface such as a shelf, counter, stair, chair, box, or stool. You should switch the foot you raise frequently from left to right. These frequent shifts will help decrease the standing stress and pressure on the lower back. For even additional stress reduction, try alternating the spread-eagle stance with the elevated foot posture.

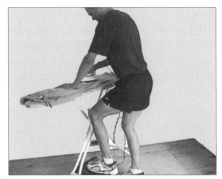

Fig. 4-7 *One foot elevated*

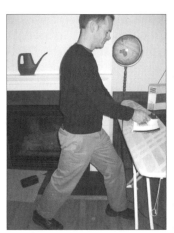

Fig. 4-8 *Try a scissor stance*

Lastly, you can try a scissor stance. Place one foot in front of the other with your feet 1-2 feet apart (Fig. 4-8). Bend the knees slightly to let the powerful leg muscles work, and to help reduce forward lean at the waist to lessen the pressure on the lower back. Frequently alternate the foot that is forward. You can try this scissor stance when ironing, cleaning and cooking, or as an alternate lifting method (see Chapter 5).

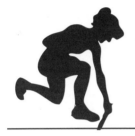

5

LIFTING

The following phone call is all too common. "I just lifted something and 'threw my back out.' I can barely get out of bed. The pain is terrible. Can you see me right now?"

When was the last time you felt lower back or neck pain after lifting something? We all do it. You lift something, even a light item, feel immediate pain, and wish you had lifted "the proper way."

The way you lift can greatly influence spinal health. Proper lifting can minimize a lot of stress on the spine. Improper lifting will accelerate wear on discs, joints and spinal tissues, and contribute to acute and chronic pain syndromes.

Bending at the waist to lift requires the postural muscles, the discs, and the joints of the lower back to bear the brunt of lifting, and places these tissues in compromised positions under a lot of pressure. The postural muscles are not designed to handle these loads, and bending forward at the waist, even if lifting a small item, places significant increases in pressure on the discs and joints (Fig. 5-1). The proper way to lift starts with spreading the feet (Fig. 5-2).

Then lift using a squat motion (Fig. 5-3) to utilize the strong *quadricep* muscles on the front of the thighs, the abdominal muscles and the rear end (*gluteal*) muscles. This squat motion protects the lower back and is much more powerful than lifting with the waist. I have seen too many patients come to my office with an acute low back pain episode which began after an improper lift, even when the load was as light as a toothbrush or pen. I always inform patients that the one bend, which was followed by sharp pain, was not the ultimate cause of the problem. The causes of the acute pain were the thousands of improper lifts previous to this single incident that accumulated spinal stress and broke down the discs, joints and muscle tissues, leading to this weakened condition. Neglecting the spine by not performing daily flexibility exercises, or through weight gain/poor diet and lack of general exercise contributes to the weakened spinal condition. An analogy I commonly use is a volcano; spinal pressure and damage builds up, unknowingly in many cases, until one last incident leads to the eruption, or causes the back to "go out." It is important to note that low back pain is a result of <u>all</u> of the improper lifts and neglect prior to the eruption.

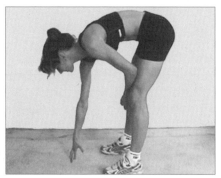

Fig. 5-1   Bending at the waist - <u>avoid</u>

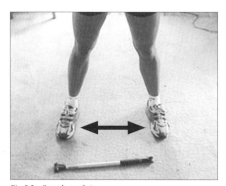

Fig. 5-2   Spread your feet

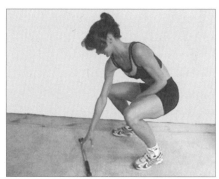

Fig. 5-3   Lift with a squat motion

There are other alternate lifting positions. Some of you have knee, hip, and other problems that may not allow this squatting position to be utilized. You could try lowering yourself onto one knee (Fig. 5-4). If you cannot perform a full squat as demonstrated, a partial squat position is much better than the typical bending at the waist lift. These proper lifting techniques should become habit, so use them with lifting any size load to become quickly accustomed to the new method.

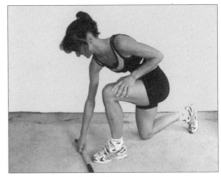

Fig. 5-4   Try lifting from one knee

Use two people whenever possible for lifting larger, bulky items and with bigger jobs. I remember one of my patients was hurt when taking a large Thanksgiving turkey out of the oven by herself. The turkey was finished cooking and no one else was around at the time to help. Her top priority was to get that turkey out of the oven so it did not overcook; however, she paid the price. I suggested next time she could leave the turkey on the open oven door or inside the oven with the oven off and plan on someone being available to help her lift it out when it is done. Avoiding a serious spinal/disc injury is more important than a slightly overcooked turkey.

It is very important, although sometimes inconvenient, to use two or more people to lift larger, oddly shaped items. When I was younger I had a construction job, and often had to take a lawnmower out of the back of a pickup truck. Lifting a mower by yourself is quite difficult and injurious. Using two people makes the lift simple, much more than twice as easy as doing it on your own! I have had numerous patients hurt themselves by lifting bulky, clumsy items like a lawnmower, air conditioner, large boxes and other items alone instead of waiting for help.

Reducing loads into smaller portions reduces spinal strain. In our high-speed lifestyles we tend to try to do things in short bursts, but the consequences can be devastating. For example, consider carrying fewer grocery bags per trip. (Try using convenient, reusable, strong, earth-friendly canvas bags.) Don't fill the wheelbarrow to the top. When moving things around the house, take lighter, more numerous trips. Be careful trying to take all of the family's laundry downstairs in one trip. (I have had patients hurt themselves this way!) If you are moving or if you are helping someone move, understand it will take time, so carry fewer items. You will thank yourself for doing so. Whenever possible, use better leverage with lifts. Take the extra moment to place yourself or the item in a more favorable position. Use tools and carriers when needed. Avoid placing bulky, heavy items low that will have to be lifted again when organizing items in your house, workplace, or shed. An often overlooked danger is moving items horizontally, such as sliding furniture along the floor or repositioning items on a table. One tends not to prepare carefully for such activities because they appear less strenuous than a full lift. Shifting of objects requires exertion and when you are unprepared it can be harmful. Again, I have had many patients hurt themselves in this avoidable way.

If you are a woman that carries a purse, empty out unnecessary, unused items. I am amazed at how heavy purses can be. Also, practice carrying a purse on the opposite shoulder, even if it feels funny, and even if the strap tends to slide off your shoulder. Carrying a purse on the same side for many years can lead to postural problems and spinal stress.

Several patients have come in hurt after picking up or playing with children. Please, take a moment to position yourself with the feet apart and use a squatting motion when lifting children. Also remember to use care when playing with children. The children may be thoroughly enjoying the game, but please don't sacrifice your spine and health. It is disheartening to see patients suffering with severe spinal pain to a point that they cannot lift and play with their children. The physical pain is compounded by the emotional anguish of being unable to do all you want or even need with children.

During some daily duties, the perfect squat position cannot be used. A good example is removing items from the trunk of your car or moving a child in or out of a car seat. When reaching into the car or taking items in and out of the trunk, try using the scissor stance (see Chapter 4). The scissor stance can be used as an alternate lifting method when items are not in locations where the spread-eagle, squat method can be used. When lifting this way, deliberately tighten your rear end and abdominal muscles for additional support. Some of the effort of the job at hand will be transferred to your rear end and legs, reducing stress on your lower back. With each lift, take an extra second or two to position yourself properly and think of how you are going to perform the lift and contract the muscles as described. I know you are busy, and may not want to be bothered with an extra few seconds of preparation, but please consider what could happen if you don't take these extra precautions. You could end up with a serious spinal problem that can adversely affect your entire life, and cost you time, pain, and money. People with "back problems" will tell you that daily pain is terrible, and consumes a tremendous amount of time in their day and interferes with everything they do; therefore, prevention is the key.

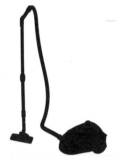

6

HOME ACTIVITIES

The frequent snowy New England winters takes its toll on backs. But your back injuries do not stop with winter. The arrival of spring brings a fresh supply of neck and back injuries from yard work and spring cleaning. Summertime gardening and pool maintenance unfortunately keeps my phone ringing from avoidable incidents. Raking leaves in the fall finishes you off.

Many patients come to my office with an episode of neck or low back pain that has followed vacuuming, shoveling snow, raking, gardening, mopping, sweeping, ironing or cleaning the house; even bending forward shaving, brushing teeth, or blow-drying hair (which also causes neck injuries). These episodes of pain are caused by poor position and posture, and changing how these activities are performed can prevent acute and chronic spinal pain syndromes. Long-handled tools such as vacuums, brooms, rakes, shovels and mops are easy to misuse and cause disc, joint and muscle stresses and pain. We tend to use these items on the same side consistently. Bending forward or to the side and pivoting at the waist when using the tools can injure (Fig. 6-1). Once again, prevention is the key, and utilizing proper positions will reduce spinal stress.

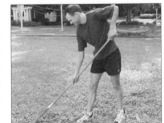

Fig. 6-1 Typical bad raking posture

VACUUMING

When using a vacuum, hold the handle with one hand and the cord (when applicable) with the other. Spread the feet apart and bend the knees somewhat in the squat position (Fig. 6-2). As you see, this is much different than the more common vacuuming position (Fig. 6-3). Rock the vacuum back and forth, controlled by the thighs, knees, feet and abs (Fig. 6-4) rather than the low back. Switch the hands on the vacuum and the cord, and make sure you split the time equally between the two sides of your body (Fig. 6-5). Obviously, one side will feel awkward at first but you will become used to it quickly. Switching hands frequently will enhance balance and distribute stress equally. When cleaning one area and reaching with the feet still, I squat low and often rest the other forearm or elbow on my leg to take additional stress off the back.

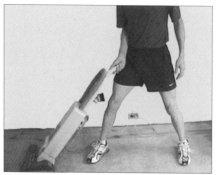

Fig. 6-2 *Spread your feet, bend your knees*

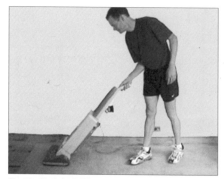

Fig. 6-3 *Typical painful vacuuming*

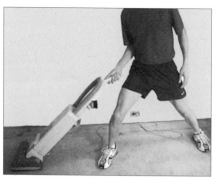

Fig. 6-4 *Use your legs, not your back*

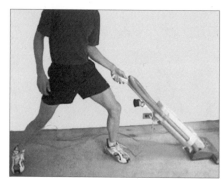

Fig. 6-5 *Try switching sides*

SHOVELING

Shoveling snow or soil requires similar changes. Bending the knees only is not enough, as you can still bend at the waist and place tremendous stress on your lower back (Fig. 6-6). Separate the feet and focus on using the quadricep (front of the thigh), gluteal (rear end), and abdominal muscles (Fig. 6-7). You can also use the arms in concert with the legs to lift and throw (Fig. 6-8). After a brief time, switch sides by changing the grip on your shovel. If you typically have your right hand low on the shovel, begin your routine with the left hand low on the shovel to make sure you use your "weak" side for half of the work, and switch frequently. This will distribute the stresses on your body evenly. It will feel odd at first to shovel on the opposite side but you will get used to it quickly and you will feel so much better after your activity. Switching sides frequently is also better for the brain (more about that in a future volume).

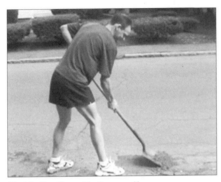

Fig. 6-6 *Shoveling and hurting yourself*

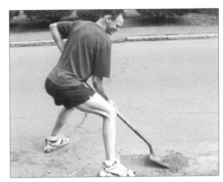

Fig. 6-7 *Spread your feet, bend your knees*

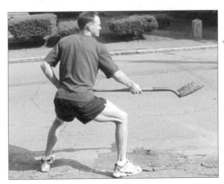

Fig. 6-8 *Throw with your arms and legs*

RAKING

Raking can cause the same disc, joint and muscle stress as shoveling and vacu-uming, so I make similar recommendations to lessen spinal stresses with this activity. The typical raking position, especially done for longer periods of time, is stressful and can lead to pain (Fig. 6-9). Instead, spread the feet comfortably apart and bend the knees. Focus the effort on the quad, gluteal, ab, and arm muscles. Use the combination of leg and arm motion to pull the rake towards you (Fig. 6-10). You can also change the stresses on your body by separating the legs apart and crouching even lower to the ground to further distribute the body stress (Fig. 6-11). Remember to put your "weak" hand low on the rake to begin, and switch to your "strong" (or usual) side after a period of time. Switch your hand positions often. Take frequent breaks and do some of the spinal stretches discussed in Chapter 2 to reduce the accumulation of spinal stress. Although the muscles in your legs may be sore by changing your raking posture, it is better to have sore legs than a damaged back!

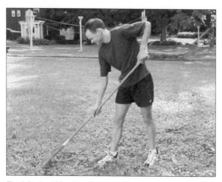

Fig. 6-9   Avoid bending at your waist

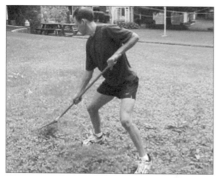

Fig. 6-10   Spread your feet, bend your knees

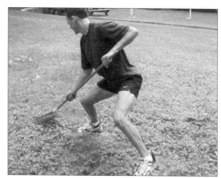

Fig. 6-11   Go lower if you can

SWEEPING

Sweeping recommendations are similar to the activities described above. A typical sweeping position can be irritating to your spine (Fig. 6-12), especially your low back. Start with an opposite hand position as you typically would and switch the hands often. Focus the work on the leg, gluteal and arm muscles (Fig. 6-13). Depending on the job and the broom, you can also take a more upright posture with both hands at the top of the broom handle (Fig. 6-14).

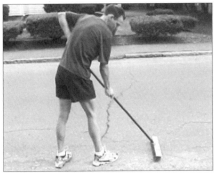

Fig. 6-12   Sweeping - avoid

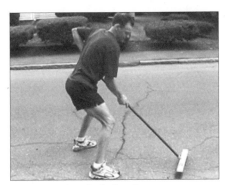

Fig. 6-13   Spread your feet, bend your knees

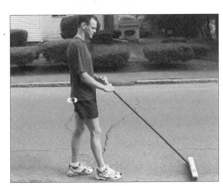

Fig. 6-14   Another good sweeping method

IRONING

Although ironing seems to be an activity that does not have the possibility to cause injury, ironing is not a "non-contact sport." Ironing for short or long periods of time can definitely apply stress and cause pain in your neck and back. Avoid the feet together, bent at the waist, chin down position (Fig. 6-15). Once again, utilize the spread-eagle position with the feet apart (Fig. 6-16) and concentrate on lifting your head as much as comfortably possible. Perhaps you have tried putting one foot up on a stool and alternating your feet (Fig. 6-17), which may be helpful. If needed, try alternating the spread-eagle and the foot-on-the-stool positions, remembering that spinal tissues thrive on motion. The more you shift and change your position, the better. For marathon ironing, take frequent breaks and undo some of the accumulation of spinal stress by doing a few of the spinal exercises discussed in Chapter 2. As another option, if you are ironing in tight quarters, try the scissor stance mentioned in Chapter 4.

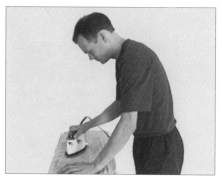

Fig. 6-15   Ironing - poor posture

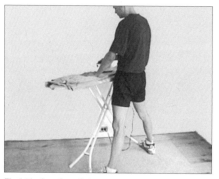

Fig. 6-16   Spread your feet

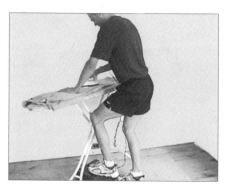

Fig. 6-17   Try one foot up and alternate

SLEEPING RECOMMENDATIONS

I am frequently asked about the best sleeping positions. I begin my answer by stating my belief: how you sleep is a minor issue as compared to how you use your body during the day. In addition, you are not in ongoing control of your sleeping position, because you are busy sleeping! However, you may be able to alter your sleep posture by starting in a less stressful position and gently and slowly training yourself to fall asleep in these positions. NOTE: Respiratory, circulatory, and neurological disorders, or significant biomechanical distortions (e.g. "widow's hump"), may prevent you from trying the following recommendations. You need to check with your healthcare practitioner.

Sleeping on your back is acceptable. However, a common mistake is sleeping on your back with one large or multiple pillows under the head and shoulders. This position will flex the head and shoulders forward (Fig. 6-18), contributing to the slumped posture we have already discussed. Avoid watching television in bed and reading in this position doing so is particularly bad for the spine. Either watch TV when lying on your stomach (provided this does not bother your lower back), or better yet, leave the television in your living room. If you sleep on your back, train yourself to sleep without a pillow, or on one thin or cervical contour pillow in order that your head will not be forced too far forward and upward. Keep in mind that any sleeping changes may take some time to get used to, so be patient. You may find that snoring will improve with these positional changes, but there are other causes of snoring (obesity, neurological dysfunction).

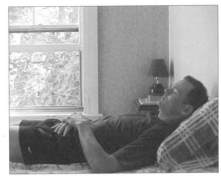

Fig. 6-18 *Sleeping - don't do this!*

Sleeping on your side can be a healthy position. Pulling the knees up towards the chest is a great way to take pressure off the spinal discs and joints, but avoid the full fetal position or C-curve with your chin tucked to your chest (Fig. 6-19). I recommend teaching yourself to lift the chin to a horizontal position in relation to the shoulders (Fig. 6-20) and avoiding the chin to chest fetal position. Try to rotate the shoulder you are laying on to the front (Fig. 6-21) instead of back (Fig. 6-22). Remember, don't force these new sleeping positions, or you may become frustrated. If you need to retreat to your old sleeping position, then do so because a full night's rest is critical for health and energy. Continue to try to make changes and slowly you can teach yourself new sleeping positions. Remember that during the night, you may unconsciously migrate back to your old sleeping position, and you may never break this habit. This is fine in my book, because what you do to yourself during the day with standing, sitting, and lifting activities is probably more injurious than what you do when you are sleeping. Plus, you may not be able to control your sleeping posture because you are busy sleeping!

Many people fall asleep on their stomach and stay that way during the night. Even though you may have been told that this is a bad position, it actually might not be bad for everyone. If you have a loss of curve in your low back (loss of the lumbar lordosis), being on your stomach puts more curve into the low back and actually may reduce disc and joint pressure. If you sleep on your stomach and enjoy a comfortable night's rest, then continue. Lying on the stomach is often combined with turning somewhat to one side or the other with one knee bent, the shoulders turned, and the head turned to one side

(Fig. 6-23). This position can be appropriate for some people. Don't worry if you cannot avoid sleeping on your stomach. Continue to get restful sleep, and a good chiropractor, physical therapist, acupuncturist, or massage therapist with a daily spinal exercise routine can clear up any ongoing spinal problems you may have.

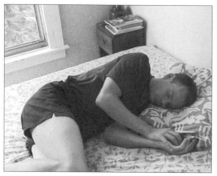
Fig. 6-19   Don't tuck the chin to the chest

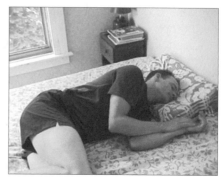
Fig. 6-20   Keep the chin level

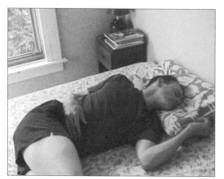
Fig. 6-21   Twisting the shoulder forward is fine

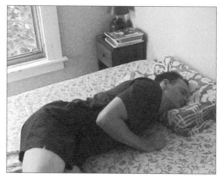
Fig. 6-22   This not as good

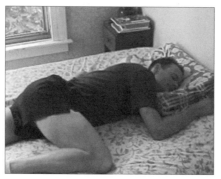
Fig. 6-23   Stomach sleepers - try this

MATTRESSES

Patients frequently ask me for recommendations about what type of mattress to buy. I begin my answer by stating that sleeping is a personal issue, and a mattress that is comfortable for one person may not be comfortable for another. A firmer mattress is generally better for most people. One way to find out if a firmer mattress is beneficial for you is to experiment by sleeping on the floor for a night. I often try this experiment with people that have acute back pain, and if you have had acute back pain, you may have already tried sleeping on the floor. Most people quickly determine if it is going to be a better night's sleep. If you find you sleep better on the floor (or on the ground when camping), a firmer mattress would probably be a better selection. If you don't, consider trying a mattress that is less firm. When shopping for a mattress, spend enough time comparing the different firmnesses. Salespeople will show you several different firmness models for comparison's sake. I also suggest trying different mattresses <u>before</u> looking at price. You may find a mid-priced mattress can serve your needs as well as a top-of-the-line model. There are mattresses on the market today that allow individual firmness adjustments from one side of the bed to the other, which may be helpful for couples. Some people I know find waterbeds provide the best night's sleep, and others like the newer memory foam styles. Again, mattress selection is a personal decision, and there is no right answer for everyone. You can also help your decision-making by noting how you sleep on hotel beds or a friend's mattress, and comparing the firmness and character of those beds to your own. Many new mattresses do not need to be flipped or turned. If you have an older mattress that should be flipped over, flip and rotate the mattress frequently, but be careful doing so and get help so you do not hurt yourself!

Finally, some people should consider a platform bed, which eliminates the box spring, allowing the mattress to rest on a wooden base. This is similar to the common activity of placing plywood between worn box springs and mattresses. It makes sense to eliminate the box spring, so the mattress is the only wearable component. As an added bonus, many platform beds have drawers underneath for storage.

PILLOWS

Which pillow is the best? This is a frequent question from my patients. My pillow recommendations are similar to mattresses. It is a personal decision, and what is successful for you may not be the answer for someone else. A smaller profile, or thinner, pillow is usually better, but unfortunately, it will be a trial-and-error experiment. There are many pillows to choose from, and they vary in size, shape, and content. Try a cervical contour pillow if you can. Many patients have enjoyed great relief from neck and arm pain, headaches, poor posture, and carpal tunnel symptoms by switching to a contour pillow. Some people prefer buckwheat pillows, while others like the "memory foam" pillows. When you find the best pillow for you, I think you will know immediately. If you are sleeping on two pillows, try one.

I consulted with a middle-aged woman several years ago who complained of bilateral wrist and hand numbness at night and especially in the morning. Although there are several possible causes of these symptoms, I asked her what position she slept in and how many pillows she was using. She explained that she usually slept on her back with two pillows under her head, so I suggested trying to sleep with only one pillow. The very next day she reported that she had no wrist or hand numbness that morning. She and I enjoyed the very easy and cheap solution.

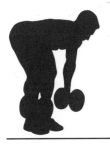

7

WEIGHTLIFTING

The next few chapters are for you, the weekend warrior and amateur athlete. I enjoy treating athletes, and helping you stay healthy and well. But, let's stay one step ahead of your injuries with a little prevention so you can continue to enjoy your choice of recreation.

Sports of all types are beneficial for overall health. If exercise selections are performed poorly, spinal stress and pain can be the result. Personally, I have significant experience regarding sports and exercise. I participated in several sports as a youth including baseball, soccer, and basketball. I started running in junior high school, and running remains a part of my life. I have competed in many road races, and completed the Boston Marathon in 2000. In 1999, I started competing in triathlons of varying distances, including half-ironman and ironman. In graduate school, I was a bodybuilder for three years, and was the training partner of a competitive bodybuilder. I have been a member of a number of gyms. Most importantly, in my chiropractic practice, I have seen a number of athletes from a large variety of sports come into my office with various complaints and spinal injuries. I have come to the realization that many of these problems can be prevented.

WEIGHTLIFTING

You have seen them at the gym. Those muscular men (and sometimes women) lifting all kinds of weight, grunting and groaning as they squeeze out that last rep with a spotter. I used to be one of them, so I'm not pointing fingers. Don't they hurt themselves working that hard? It looks like some of them are "cheating," using other muscles and body movements as they lift too much weight. This can be dangerous.

As I discussed in Chapter 1, the most important factors for a healthy lower back are <u>not</u> muscle strength and size of the back muscles. I see many people with extremely strong back muscles who still suffer from lower back pain. Therefore, I do not recommend low back extensor muscle exercises for most people, especially dead lifts. Remember, the main issue for a healthy spine is flexibility, not strength. As always, an excellent time to perform the spinal flexibility exercises (Chapter 2) is before and after workouts.

As I make my recommendations regarding weightlifting, I realize if you are a bodybuilder and lift weights as your primary exercise routine, you may not adhere to these recommendations. I have seen a number of injuries resulting from weightlifting, both machine and free weights, that could have been prevented by avoiding certain exercises, modifying others, and replacing more dangerous exercises with safer ones. Although I do not lift weights with bodybuilding intensity any longer, I still consistently do weight workouts. The difference now is I lift to maintain tone, to vary my workouts (cross-train), and to try to minimize injuries from my other activities. Now I lift much lighter weights; each repetition and motion is much slower; I pay much more attention to posture and form; and I keep the repetitions of each set much higher. With many exercises, the amount of weight I lift now is half of what I lifted in the past, and the repetitions have doubled.

Proper form and posture when lifting weights is critical in reducing spinal and joint stress, and to help prevent injuries. I recommend that certain exercises be avoided completely and other exercises be modified to reduce spinal stress. Again, I realize if you are a serious bodybuilder or personal trainer, you may not agree with my list of exercises to avoid. I am relaying my experience with patients who seek care for injuries resulting from weight lifting incidents. The exercises that most commonly cause injuries are included in the list below.

EXERCISES TO AVOID

These are some of the exercises to avoid (Figures 7-1 through 7-12). Any exercise requiring the weights to be placed behind the head such as pull-downs, military presses, and tricep extensions should be avoided. These exercises require your head to be flexed forward in relationship to your upper body while you are exerting significant effort, and this places tremendous stresses on the discs, joints, and muscles of your cervical spine (neck). Additionally, the behind-the-head pull-down puts the shoulder and elbow in vulnerable positions, which can injure these joints.

EXERCISES TO AVOID

Seated back extension (7-1)	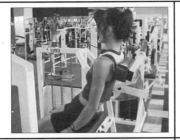	Dead lift (7-7)	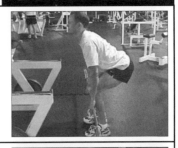
Behind-the-head pull-down (7-2)	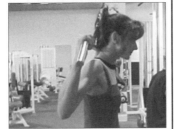	Squats (unless strict and very light) (7-8)	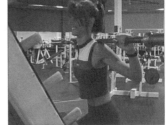
Behind-the-head shoulder press (7-3)	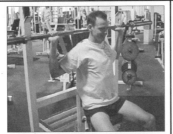	Lunges (unless strict and light) (7-9)	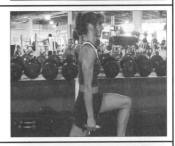
Behind-the-head tricep extension (7-4)	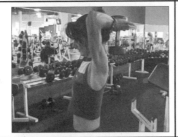	Clean and jerk (7-10)	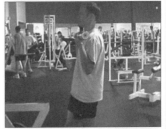
Bent-over row (7-5)	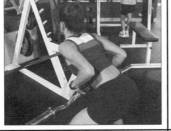	Good morning (unless strict and light) (7-11)	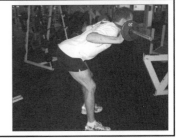

Seated row (unless strict and light) (7-6)	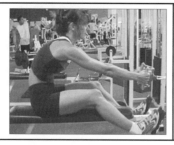	Upright row (7-12)	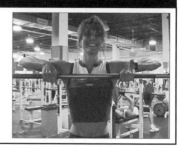

One of the most important recommendations I can make in regard to all weightlifting exercises, whether you use free weights or machines, is to keep your head up and your chin higher. Take a moment to observe people at your gym: most of them will have their chin and head positioned downward (unless they have read this book or they have a personal trainer who has taught them proper positioning). Lifting your head and keeping your chin up at least horizontal (Fig. 7-13) may take some time getting used to but this is important so stay with it. I have had many patients come to me with acute neck,

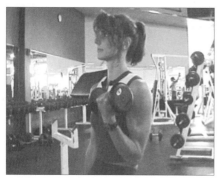

Fig. 7-13 Keep your chin level at all times

shoulder, and arm pain resulting from behind-the-head exercises, or having the head forward and chin down during other exercises. I recall one patient who came in for treatment with acute neck pain on two different occasions after doing tricep dips with his chin pulled down to his chest (Fig. 7-14). Although I showed him the safe head position (Fig. 7-14A) after the first episode, he did not change his ways until he painfully re-learned the lesson after the second injury.

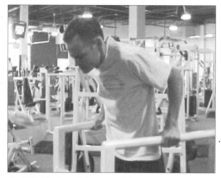

Fig. 7-14 Do this and you are asking for trouble

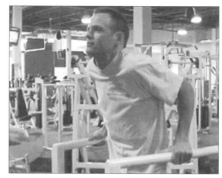

Fig. 7-14A This is better

Squats, dead lifts, bent-over rows, clean and jerk and other similar exercises place tremendous stresses on the lower back discs and joints. Squats with weights over the back of the shoulders increase neck stress, and squats and lunges place a lot of stress on the knees. Many of you will disagree with this recommendation, as we all have been taught that squats are one of the best overall strength and size building exercise one can do, and squats were a major focus for me back in my bodybuilding days. Are the added neck, low back, and knee stresses and injuries worth it if you are not a competitive bodybuilder? Those wishing to decrease the possibility of injury can replace squats and lunges with effective, safer substitutes. Knee extension and leg press machines will more safely build the quadriceps and other muscle groups, while reducing spinal stress. Toe raises and leg curls will effectively target the calf and hamstring muscle groups. If you are having knee problems, consider using much lighter weight and increasing repetitions with the knee extension and leg press exercises to reduce additional knee stress. Follow the advice of your physical therapist or trainer regarding specific exercises and positions for your knee rehabilitation. Typically, those who are using weights for knee rehab are already using lighter weights and slower repetitions.

There are numerous other back-building exercises that can replace bent-over rows and behind-the-head pull-downs, including my favorite, which is wide grip pull-downs to the chest with the chin up (Fig. 7-15). One-arm rows (Fig. 7-16) and many back machines (Fig. 7-17) can replace the behind-the-neck pull-downs or unsupported two-hand bent-over rows. Seated rows should be avoided unless they are performed with light weights and very strict form (Figures 7-18 and 7-18A), but I do not do this exercise any longer due to injury potential. A seated row machine with a chest pad is much safer (and don't forget to keep your chin up). Remember, with any exercise you perform, keep the chin level or slightly up. As a simple example, consider the bicep curl in Figures 7-19 & 7-20. The curl in Fig. 7-19 shows a bicep curl head position that you will frequently see in the gym. You will notice many people with their head down as they are looking at the action of the exercise, instead of looking straight ahead. Figure 7-20 shows the safer way of performing a bicep curl.

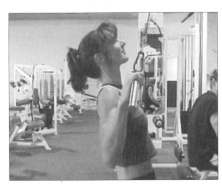

Fig. 7-15   A safe lat pulldown

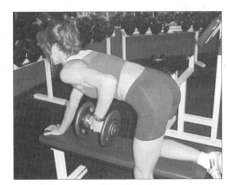

Fig. 7-16   One arm row - chin up, flat back

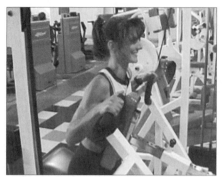

Fig. 7-17   Keep the chin level

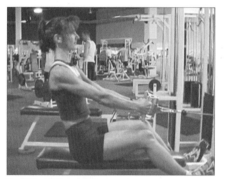

Fig. 7-18   A Safer seated row

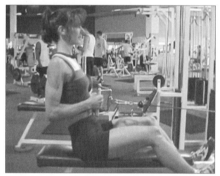

Fig. 7-18A   Be careful of your lower back

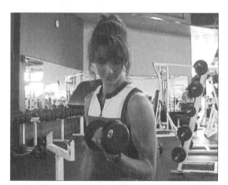

Fig. 7-19   Don't look at your weights

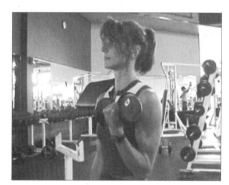

Fig. 7-20   Always the keep the chin level

There are many options for tricep exercises; therefore, behind-the-head tricep extensions are not necessary. The behind-the-head shoulder press (military press) can be replaced by shoulder presses in front of the head and face (Fig. 7-21), and with other shoulder exercises and machines. If you are not fluent in the many exercises available for each muscle group, a personal trainer or physical therapist can show you a variety of safer replacements for each muscle group.

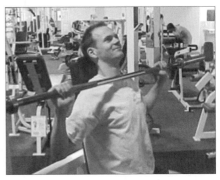

Fig. 7-21   Keep shoulder presses to the front

IMPROVING POSTURE WITH WEIGHTS

A few recommendations are very beneficial for the spine and posture of most people. Make sure your physical therapist or healthcare practitioner approves these exercises before you begin. Many people suffer from poor posture as they age (Fig. 7-22), with rounded shoulders, a forward head shift, and an increased curve in the middle back. This poor posture results from many years of a slouching posture and from the front muscles on the upper body (chest, biceps) having greater tone and development than

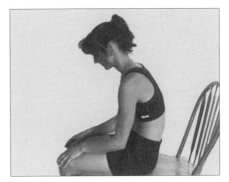

Fig. 7-22   Let's try to avoid this

the muscles on the back of the body (back, triceps, spinal postural muscles). The muscles of your upper back and the smaller postural muscles typically lose strength from neurological changes as compared to the muscles in the front of the torso. The exercise selections you make with weights, and your posture during exercising and daily activities can greatly influence your posture and long-term spinal (and overall) health. You can assist your body in maintaining a more upright posture by doing more back and tricep exercises and fewer chest and bicep exercises. Many find it easier to build chest and bicep muscles as compared to back and tricep muscles, and often chest and bicep exercises receive more focus, which perpetuates poor posture. Again, for those of you that are not competitive bodybuilders, consider doing two sets of back, tricep, and shoulder exercises for every one set of chest and bicep exercises. If the 2:1 ratio seems too odd, consider a ratio of three to two when comparing the number of back and tricep exercises to chest and bicep exercises. For instance, on weeks that I work out with weights three times, I will do two back, tricep, and shoulder workouts as compared to one chest and bicep workout. On days when I do a full body workout, I will do two back, tricep, and shoulder sets for every set of chest and biceps. This promotes a more upright posture by increasing strength of the muscles that work against slouching.

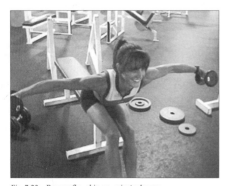
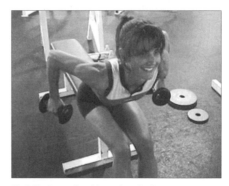

Fig. 7-23   *Reverse fly - chin up - ninety degress*   Fig. 7-24   *Reverse fly - chin up - forty-five degress*

There are specific exercises I recommend trying to help fight your slouching posture, and to help balance the back-to-front muscle groups. Try a reverse fly with very light weight at ninety degrees and a little heavier at forty-five degrees (Figures 7-23 & 7-24). Also, try one-arm rows, which are at zero degrees when comparing the relationship of the arm to the body (Fig. 7-16). If you have shoulder problems, please use extra care when trying these exercises. Start with very light weights, go slowly and keep your chin up and shoulders back as shown in the pictures. Some of you might even want to start with no weight to understand the motion and see how you feel. You will probably notice the ninety-degree reverse fly requires lighter weights than the forty-five degree reverse fly. Personally, I use 10-12 pounds for the ninety-degree reverse fly and 12-15 pounds for the forty-five degree reverse fly. Stronger people can use heavier weight, and some of you who are just beginning may have to use extremely light weight, perhaps as light as two or three pounds.

Regarding the amount of weight to use, I always mention I would rather see you start too easy and light rather than too hard. Many people, especially those returning to workouts after some time off, tend to start too hard and heavy, which often leads to injuries. Remember, if you start "too" easy, you can always increase weight, repetitions, and sets on another day, as long as you are able to maintain proper posture and form as discussed. If you start too hard, you can't take it back. Starting too hard could lead to more time off, and you may need the services of a chiropractor or other health care professional for injuries. I also recommend chiropractic wellness checkups and adjustments for weightlifters and other athletes. It is easier and cheaper to keep you well than it is to fix you when you are broken.

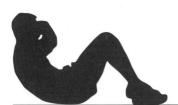

8

ABDOMINALS

Many people desire flat stomachs and well-defined abdominal muscles. However, the main keys to "ripped" abdominals are proper eating habits and cardiovascular exercise, both of which are commonly ignored. Proper eating habits include avoiding processed food and eating more vegetables and fruit. I recommend modeling your food selections after what most of the thin, disease-free people around the world eat. Low fat, high energy, healthy plant foods are the main staples of a healthy diet, and they include complex carbohydrates (beans, yams, sweet potatoes, rice (except short grain white rice), oats, and other non-processed whole grains), and lots of varied vegetables and fruit. High calorie, saturated fat animal foods (beef, chicken, seafood, dairy products and eggs) and pro-cessed foods with hydrogenated and trans-fats will keep weight on and hide your washboard abs with a layer of fat. Time and time again I hear about people wishing that they had a flat stomach who engage in intense ab work-outs, but become frustrated. In many cases after the intense ab program, the ab muscles become very well developed but remain hidden under a layer of fat. Moreover, some people develop back and neck pain as a result of the strenu-ous abdominal exercises. Let me emphasize the most important thing, which is to eat more calorie-dilute healthier plant foods, while significantly reducing or eliminating processed snack foods and soda. The second most important thing is to engage in cardiovascular exercise to burn more calories (under the guidance of a qualified interested healthcare practitioner).

Let me remind you that we cannot "spot reduce." This means if you have a particular area of your body such as your stomach, rear-end, or legs, that has excess fat you want to lose, you cannot lose it by only exercising that singular body part. This is why those that do only ab workouts to shed unwanted fat in the stomach area are usually frustrated with the results. To lose unwanted fat in select trouble spots, you need to work your total body. Remember, the most important thing is to eat fewer calories (increase calorie dilute foods and reduce calorie dense foods as I mentioned) and the second most important thing is to do regular cardiovascular workouts. Yes, you can tone and tighten a particular area with targeted exercises, but you cannot "spot reduce" fat.

Many of you are already involved with intense ab workouts and have had results. I understand that some of you will disagree with the following comments and may not follow my recommendations. Those of you who want to protect your lower back and neck from injury, and at the same time perform excellent abdominal exercise, might want to try these recommendations. Many ab exercises can be harmful to your lower back and neck. Many patients come to my office with acute neck and back pain resulting from harmful ab exercises. After taking my advice and stopping their ab exercise program, many patients notice their neck and back complaints begin to improve immediately. I am not saying you can never do any abdominal exercises. As a replacement, I recommend a modified crunch exercise. You may not think this is enough intensity for your abdominals, but in my experience these crunches will offer an intense ab workout, with the benefit of protecting your spine from injury.

These are the ab exercises I recommend. Place your legs on a table, chair, bench or bed (Fig. 8-1). Pull your knees close to your chest so that the angle between your knees and stomach is less than ninety degrees (Fig. 8-2). This position flattens out the low back curve, extends the pelvis backwards, and takes significant stress off the lumbar discs and joints. This position also eliminates leg muscles from the exercise, isolating the abs. You can place your hands be-

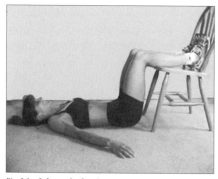

Fig. 8-1 Safe crunch - Step 1

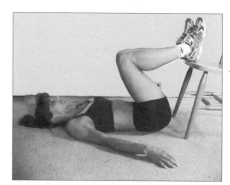

Fig. 8-2 Safe crunch - Step 2

hind your head to support the weight of your head (Fig. 8-3), but do not pull on your head. The relationship between your head and ribcage should remain unchanged during the crunch (Fig. 8-4), so do not pull your chin to your chest. A good way to envision this exercise is imagine a string attached to the center of your chest which pulls your upper body toward the ceiling.

Twist from side to side to work the oblique abdominal muscles first (Fig. 8-5). You can then perform straight-up crunches to work the rectus abdominal muscles (Fig. 8-4). I recommend doing more of the twisting oblique crunches and less of the straight up rectus crunches. The oblique abdominal muscles are more involved in torso and low back stabilization as compared to the rectus abdominal muscles. Consider working the abs no more often than every other day as these skeletal muscles benefit from rest just like any other muscle group, but you can work your abs daily if the sets and repetitions are not excessive. Currently I do one set of oblique crunches and one set of straight rectus crunches each day, with each set consisting of 25-50 repetitions. Again I know some of you prefer doing hundreds of crunches instead of only 50, but this system, coupled with improved food intake and regular cardiovascular exercise will get most of you the flat, defined abs you are looking for.

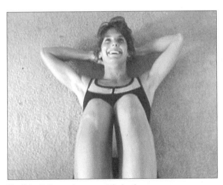

Fig. 8-3   Safe crunch - support the head

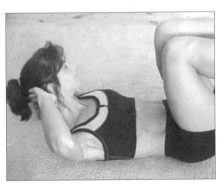

Fig. 8-4   Safe crunch - straight up

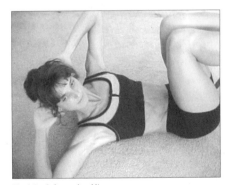

Fig. 8-5   Safe crunch - obliques

Please notice as you perform these crunches how little you have to raise your upper body off the floor to get an efficient workout and feel the burn (Figures 8-6 and 8-7). If you want more intensity you can simply perform more repetitions and more sets of these exercises. Another way to increase the intensity is to hold your body in the crunched position for a second or two.

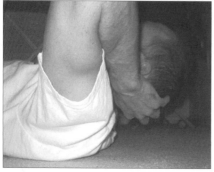 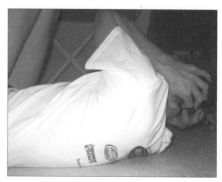

Fig. 8-6   Safe crunch - don't come up too far   *Fig. 8-7   Safe crunch - oblique*

This method of ab work isolates the abdominal muscles and leaves leg muscles out of the picture. Many other ab exercises such as ramp boards, leg raises, ab machines, and knee-ups will recruit hip flexor muscles during the motion, pulling on the lower back discs. These exercises also increase low back disc pressure, which could lead to irritation and pain. Strengthening the hip flexors may lead to lower back problems. The iliopsoas muscle, a strong hip flexor, actually has attachments to the low back discs. Some of you with existing lower back problems might have already found out that abdominal exercises such as knee-ups and leg raises increase your pain. Many people already have an increased lumbar curve (lordosis) and strengthening hip flexors such as the iliopsoas could increase the curve further and lead to more problems. Many of my patients gain quick relief from lower back pain with elimination of knee-ups, ramp board, leg raises, and ab machine exercises. In rare cases, some people with a loss of curve in their lower back find that these ab exercises actually relieves their lower back pain. Because each of you have different structures and needs, it is best to consult with a chiropractor, therapist, or trainer familiar with exercise and your individual condition to determine which exercises are best for your spine. If you stop your ab program, but still have back and neck pain, consider an evaluation by a chiropractor.

Please remember the secrets to a flat stomach and developed abdominals. Eliminate processed foods and soda, decrease animal foods, while increasing vegetable, fruit, and whole grain foods. Also, increase your cardiovascular exercise to burn more calories and fat. These are excellent recommendations in general, and you will be thrilled with the results.

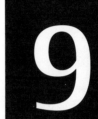

9

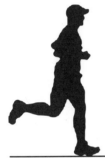

WALKING, JOGGING AND RUNNING

A s a runner since junior high school I have had the opportunity to observe the postures of many runners, walkers and joggers. For simplicity's sake, during the following discussion I will use the word runner, which will include runners, joggers and walkers. I would like to make one simple, yet very important recommendation. If your running posture is improved you may become more efficient and faster. You also may avoid additional spinal stresses, especially in the neck, upper mid-back, and lower back. A typical running posture has the arms in front of the chest, rocking in an angular side-to-side motion in relation to the direction of travel (Fig. 9-1). Consider improving this arm motion by placing the arms along the side of the body. Rock the arms at the shoulder joint in a forward and backward manner, along the path of travel (Fig. 9-2). The weight and force of the arm swing will now be directed straight ahead, which is much more efficient than crossing the arms in front. Please observe that the improper oblique arm swing uses unnecessary energy as the body is trying to move forward and the arms are trying to rotate and pull the body to the side. For another example of the efficient form, observe sprinters. They tend to exaggerate the straight forward and backward swing of the arms for maximum speed and efficiency (Fig. 9-3). The improvement in the arm swing can be learned by making sure the bent elbow is drawn backwards as far as comfortably possible (Fig. 9-4). Imagine that someone is grabbing your elbow and pulling it straight back. Be patient, remembering that forming this new habit will take time and conscious effort and you may find yourself slipping back into your old running posture at times. Even after making this change myself over several years, I find that I have to concentrate on drawing the elbows backward while running. The improvements to your posture, spine and running efficiency will be worth this extra effort.

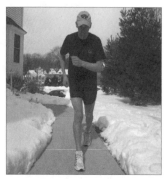

Fig. 9-1   Avoid arms crossing midline

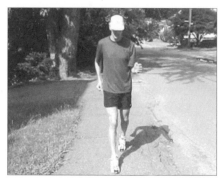

Fig. 9-2   Swing the arms straight ahead

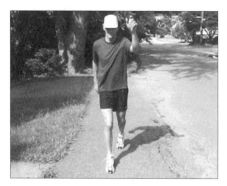

Fig. 9-3   Bigger arm swing for speed

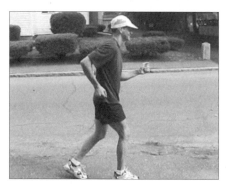

Fig. 9-4   Pull the elbow straight back

Other improvements can be made to the walking, jogging, and running form. Pulling your shoulders backwards to create a more upright posture will assist the proper arm swing (Fig. 9-5), and decrease the rounding of the middle back and ribcage. The improved posture also expands the ribcage allowing for greater lung capacity and increased oxygen uptake. This posture recommendation echoes the good general posture instructions I make throughout this book. Try lifting your chin somewhat to decrease the forward head position and look downward with your eyes to watch the ground.

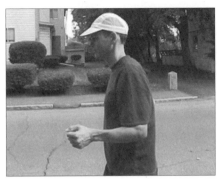

Fig. 9-5   Keep the shoulders back

In review, swinging the arms straight along the side, pulling the shoulders backward and lifting the chin will improve the efficiency of your workout and reduce spinal stresses in the neck, upper mid-back and low back. If you have postural problems you can't seem to correct on your own, consider having an evaluation by a chiropractor. You will learn posture-improving exercises, and chiropractic adjustments may help.

For general healthy advice, and to create new healthy habits, I recommend doing a set of the warm-up spinal exercises described in Chapter 2 before and after your runs and walks. A set of these spinal stretches (which take only one minute) before your workout warms the spine up in preparation for it, and a set after your workout helps decrease the accumulation of spinal stress.

Exercise smart. If you are new to exercise, or getting back into it after an extended break, don't go too hard, too soon.

How can you monitor your intensity and progress, and work out more efficiently? Try a heart rate monitor, and use the information from Sally Edward's website, Heartzones.com.

10

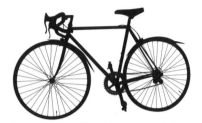

CYCLING

The popular hybrid and mountain bikes tend to promote a more up-right position, so not much can be changed to help improve the riding posture. You can still slouch on hybrids and mountain bikes, so be aware of your posture and try to keep from hunching over. The road bike position has riders slouched and curled up for long periods. When on training rides, consider changing the crouched position as much as the work-out will permit, even off the "hoods" (top of the brake levers). Change position frequently between the drops, hoods, and the top of the handlebars when-ever possible, to help reduce neck, mid-back, low back and abdominal organ stress. This recommendation may not work for some of you during intense workout and race situations, however, you may still want to consider coming out of the crouched racing posture from time to time during longer races. I once read a story of an ironman triathlete who had to have abdominal surgery after a Hawaiian Ironman Triathlon due to a lack of blood flow to abdominal organs during the bike section of the race. One of the reasons this may have occurred is that blood flow is diverted from the abdominal area to the legs due to the demands put on the body. Another factor is the sustained crouched bike posture, particularly the "aero" or "time trial" position, which can create additional abdominal pressure and squeeze blood from the area. Dehydration could have been an added problem. I realize in a race situation every second

₋unts, especially at that level of competition, but I also believe people need to consider their future health.

In addition to changing positions frequently during rides, I have found some stretches to be beneficial to reduce neck, upper back, and lower back strain. Like many other riders I tend to suffer from some neck and upper back tension during longer rides, but these stretches reduce some discomfort. With my hands in the drops, hoods, or on the top crossbar of the handlebar, I will push my upper back up through the shoulders and lift my head up (Fig. 10-1). I will then allow my middle back and head to fall down in between my shoulders (Fig. 10-2), holding each position for a few seconds, and repeat several times. This will stretch out the neck, upper traps and upper back and interrupt the constant static position to help improve blood flow and tissue motion. In addition, you can stretch the middle and lower back by doing a "cat-cow" stretch during cycling. Start off by accentuating the curves in your middle and lower back like a cat raising the hair on its back (Fig. 10-3). Then, stick out your abdomen and flatten out the middle back for the "cow" portion of the stretch (Fig. 10-4). As always, consider doing a set of the spinal flexibility exercises in Chapter 2 before and after bike workouts to stretch the spinal discs, joints, and muscles, and to help decrease the accumulation of spinal stress. Remember, these spinal stretches only take a minute to complete. If you are a recreational or competitive cyclist, consider a chiropractic evaluation to deal with any existing spinal aches and pains, improve your posture, and to help prevent future problems.

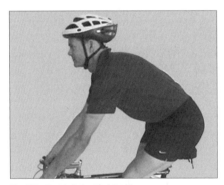

Fig. 10-1   *Stretch the head and shoulders up*

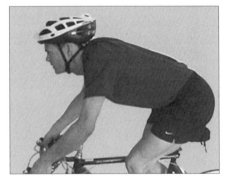

Fig. 10-2   *Stretch the head and shoulders down*

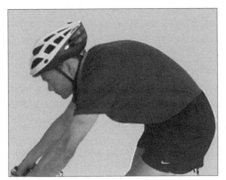

Fig. 10-3   Cat stretch

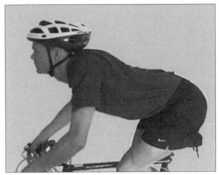

Fig. 10-4   Cow stretch

People frequently ask me what kind of exercise is best for their children. Anything is better than nothing! Any exercise is better than TV, computers, and computer games!

For brain development, exercise requiring more difficult coordination may be better. I like ping-pong (especially with the non-dominant hand), jump rope, swimming, martial arts (without intense sparring), and cross-country skiing, among other sports.

11

SWIMMING

S wimming is a wonderful exercise selection for many people, with excellent cardiovascular benefits, muscle toning of all major muscle groups, and low joint stress. Swimming is not for everyone as pools and temperate fresh and salt water are not accessible to all, and chlorine exposure is a concern. The muscle toning and strengthening can be enhanced with certain swimming drills and exercises. There are many excellent exercise and aerobic classes in pools nowadays, even yoga. Swimming greatly reduces spinal stresses as compared to other types of exercise selections. If you swim in indoor or outdoor pools that are treated with chlorine, you may consider increasing your salt (NaCl) intake to counteract the effects of increased chlorine in your system. Please only do this under the advice of your physician and avoid if you have sensitivity to salt due to certain medical conditions.

If you have been swimming for a long time, you may find this next recommendation difficult or impossible. However, if you are relatively new to swimming you may have more success. When doing the crawl (freestyle), consider training yourself to rotate your head and breathe on both sides of your body as opposed to only one side. This will reduce neck stress and possible abnormal postures and neurological problems. Breathing on both sides will symmetrically stimulate your vestibular system (balance/cerebellum areas of your brain). When I began to swim in 1998 I trained myself to breathe on both sides, and I am able to do so comfortably now. I do have a stronger side, therefore, on training swims I focus on breathing more with the "weak" side. When racing, I breathe more on the stronger side. In other words, I "train my weakness and race my strength." Several experienced swimmers tell me they cannot breathe on both sides, and it may be too late to change. It is worth attempting even if you have been swimming for a long period of time. You can treat breathing on your weak or opposite side as a new challenge to your workout and you can spend some portion of workouts breathing only on your weak side. Please consult with your healthcare practitioner before making these changes, and if you begin to breathe on your opposite side and feel symptoms of dizziness or lightheadedness, stop immediately and consult him or her.

There are other hazards with swimming, particularly diving. Dr. Michael Gazdar, DC, CCSP, in his book *Taking Your Back To The Future*[8], talks about Greg Louganis in the 1988 Olympics. He hit the back of his head on the platform during the diving competition. He went to the team chiropractor, Dr. Jan Corwin of Oakland, CA, and received an adjustment of his cervical spine. Greg then went on to win a goal medal in that event. Swimmers and other athletes regularly receive chiropractic care not only for injuries, but to achieve top performance potential.

DIZZINESS

Those of you with dizziness, equilibrium problems, or vertigo during swimming or any other activity, especially if the cause has not been identified or treatment has not been successful, should consider chiropractic as a treatment option. Chiropractors and chiropractic neurologists have successfully treated many patients with dizziness conditions. Personally I have had several patients respond well to conservative chiropractic care for their equilibrium problems. Dizziness, vertigo, and equilibrium problems can have various causes including cerebellum dysfunctions, vestibular-based problems, BPPV (*Benign Paroxysmal Positional Vertigo*), and cervical spine dysfunctions and subluxations. Obviously, swimmers with dizziness problems have great trouble returning to workouts before the cause of their dizziness has been identified and corrected. If you suffer from dizziness or vertigo, you should consider consultation with a healthcare practitioner familiar with the diagnosis and treatment of these disorders, including chiropractors and chiropractic neurologists.

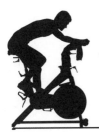

12

CARDIOVASCULAR
EXERCISE EQUIPMENT

Concentration on improving your posture when using cardiovascular equipment can significantly reduce spinal stress. The treadmill posture should follow the same recommendations as I made in the Chapter 9, Walking, Jogging, and Running. When using a stair stepper machine, please consider not leaning forward with your arms resting on the machine for long periods (Fig. 12-1). Try to utilize the upright position as much as possible (Fig. 12-2), although switching frequently and spending brief periods in the slouched position is fine. On cross-trainer or elliptical machines the same upright posture should be utilized with the chin-up and shoulders drawn back (Fig. 12-3), as opposed to a chin-down, slouched posture (Fig. 12-4). If you use a UBE (upper body ergometer), assume an upright posture with the chin up and shoulders drawn back (Fig. 12-5), instead of a slouched, chin-down posture (Fig. 12-6).

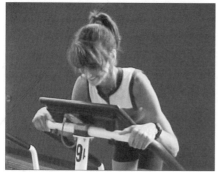

Fig. 12-1   Step machine - don't do this for long periods

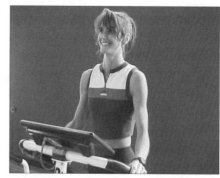

Fig. 12-2   Step machine - better posture

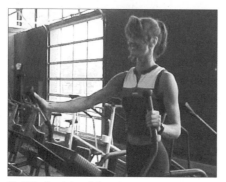

Fig. 12-3   Crosstrainer - better posture

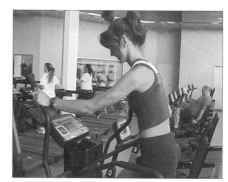

Fig. 12-4   Crosstrainer - try to avoid

It appears to be easy to misuse rowing machines as a slouched posture with reaching and leaning forward too far is easy to do (Fig. 12-7). Consider not leaning forward as much during the relaxation phase of rowing (Fig. 12-8) and pull yourself to an upright, erect posture during the pull phase of the stroke. Accentuate the upright posture by pushing your chest and ribcage out in front of you during the pull phase of the movement, which will help counteract the slouching tendency. Keep the arms beside your body and focus on pulling the elbows a bit further backward, which will increase the workload on the back muscles for additional benefit. As with all other posture recommendations, try to keep the chin up and shoulders back as much as possible to reduce spinal stresses during exercise.

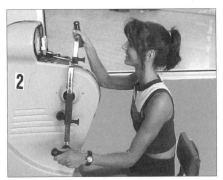

Fig. 12-5 UBE - correct

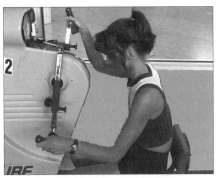

Fig. 12-6 UBE - incorrect

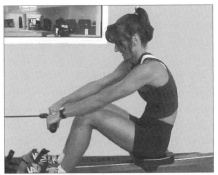

Fig. 12-7 Rowing machine - incorrect

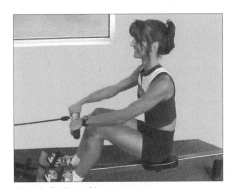

Fig. 12-8 Rowing machine - correct

When using upright or recumbent bicycles, concentrate on keeping the shoulders back and chin up. If you read during exercise on either of these bikes, it is easy to fall into a slouched posture (Figures 12-9 and 12-10). Either consider not reading, or holding what you are reading higher (Figures 12-11 and 12-12). If you read on the bike, consider taking breaks to stretch back, and even do the spinal extension exercise on the bike (Figures 12-13 and 12-14). You can vary positions on the upright bike from a straight-up position (Fig. 12-15), to hands on the bars (Fig. 12-16) to the "aero" position (Fig. 12-17). Many of you have already noticed frequent shifting of position helps dissipate spinal stress. As always, a good habit to form is to do the spinal flexibility exercises (Chapter 2) before and after cardiovascular workouts. It only takes a minute to do these stretches, and the benefits can last a lifetime!

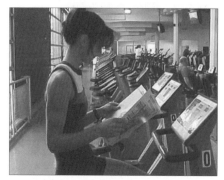
Fig. 12-9   Upright bike - avoid

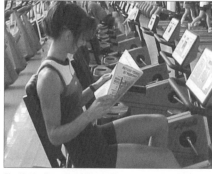
Fig. 12-10   Recumbent bike - avoid

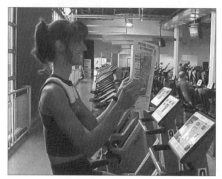
Fig. 12-11   Upright bike - better

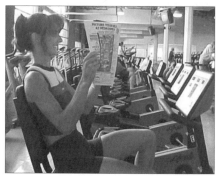
Fig. 12-12   Recumbent bike - better

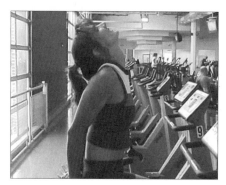
Fig. 12-13   Upright bike - spinal extension

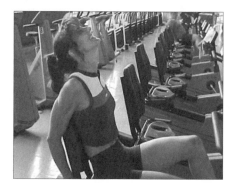
Fig. 12-14   Recumbent bike - spinal extension

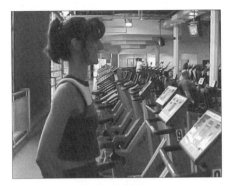

Fig. 12-15   Upright bike - hands off the bars

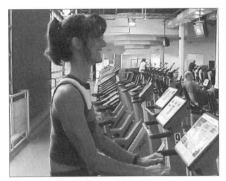

Fig. 12-16   Upright bike - hands on bars

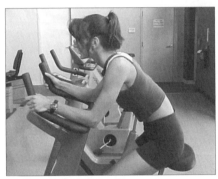

Fig. 12-17   Upright bike - aero position

Keys to injury-free golf:

1. *Do the spinal warm-ups in chapter 2 after getting up in the morning and when you get to the course, before you start swinging.*

2. *Don't grab the driver and start with full-intensity swings. Start with a low iron, chip shot warm-ups, and gradually build intensity.*

3. *Don't try to hurt the ball. Your back may not like you.*

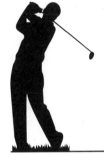

13

GOLF

olf is considered less physically demanding than other sports, but due to its unique nature, injuries are relatively common. Many injuries result from improper warm-up, swinging too hard, and abrupt stoppage of a swing by the club striking something. Other injuries are a result of accumulation of stresses because the golf swing is asymmetrical, which applies unbalanced forces on the body. I have treated many golfers in my clinic and have seen consistent injuries, particularly in the lower back, due to the reasons described above. I have golfed over many years so I have a first-hand understanding of the forces and traumas involved with this sport.

One recommendation I consistently make to reduce golf injury is appropriate warm-up. Before you leave your house to get to the golf course, start with the warm-up exercises described in Chapter 2. This will begin preparing the discs, joints and muscles of your spine and body for the demands of golf. When arriving at the course consider doing another set of the exercises especially if it has been a lengthy car ride. Please avoid what many golfers do, which is go to the first tee, pull the driver out of the bag, and start swinging at full intensity. Instead, start your swing warm-up with a smaller iron such as a wedge. Swing this iron side to side equally and easily as if you were using a weed whacker. Start the swinging slowly with low intensity. Do this 10-20 times per side, building up the amount and intensity of the swing as you proceed. Next, practice chipping for 20 seconds. Build this up to a half-swing, then a full swing when you feel warm and ready. At the first tee consider the same warm-up procedure with the driver as you did with the iron. Swing the driver side to side as if using a weed whacker, starting with a low intensity and small swing size. Increase the speed, intensity and range of the swing after several strokes. Start with quarter swings, then progress to half swings and then to a full swing with full speed when you feel ready. This warm-up activity will only take a minute or two, but may prevent unnecessary stress and injury to your spine, and avoidable time off from golf. Throughout the round you can always perform these stretching exercises as you see fit.

A golf instructor once told me some advice that he commonly tells students, and it is advice I frequently pass along. He said, "Don't try to hurt the ball." I absolutely agree with this recommendation. The intensity of the swing can influence injury potential. As swing intensity increases, stress and injury to the discs, joint ligaments and other soft tissues in and around the spine increase as well. Consider decreasing the intensity and power you put into your swing to decrease the accumulation of spinal stresses. As an added benefit, many golfers have observed that when they decreased swing intensity, their accuracy and score improved. Work on developing a smooth complete swing with a little less intensity and you may find that your game actually improves.

There are other swing modifications that may be considered to decrease spinal stress and injury. A golf instructor and other golfers have all recommended that I slow down my back swing, which keeps the swing itself under better control. Slowing down the back swing will decrease spinal stress and torque, therefore decreasing the amount of force and injury potential on the spine. If you focus on making solid consistent contact with the ball instead of trying to out-drive the other players and tear the ball's cover off, you will significantly reduce the spinal stress when playing golf.

In review, there are several things that you can do to decrease spinal stress during golf. Perform your spinal exercises as described in Chapter 2 before leaving home, and another set when you arrive at the course. Instead of starting to swing at 100% effort with your driver, begin with a small iron and swing side to side equally to warm up the tissues in and around your spine. Slowly and gradually build up the effort of your swing and take a minute with the iron before you start to swing your driver. Please try not to "hurt the ball." These recommendations will help decrease accumulations of spinal stress and the likelihood of injury. Consider being evaluated by a chiropractor well before you have pain or an injury in an effort to improve your overall spinal health and flexibility, and perhaps even your golf game itself. As many of you may know, several professional golfers have personal chiropractors and even take them to tournaments!

14

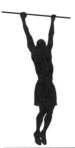

ADVANCED
SPINAL EXERCISES

I n clinical practice I am continuously challenged on ways to motivate people to follow through with the spinal flexibility exercises in Chapter 2. Many of you are willing and eager to do more to improve your spinal and overall health, and there are many other activities and exercises you can try. A few of them are described here. As always, please try these exercises under the guidance of your own healthcare professional, and ask your doctor or therapist if these exercises are appropriate for your particular condition. There are other excellent, healthy options to consider that many find beneficial, including yoga, pilates, and martial arts for you to try.

BALANCE/SWISS BALLS

These large, light, inflatable balls are becoming more and more popular in physical therapy offices, chiropractic offices and gymnasiums. If you are using a balance ball for the first time, please get guidance on which exercises are appropriate and be sure to start slowly and safely. These balls can provide excellent rehabilitation for your spine and nervous system. Ball activities will help strengthen and stabilize postural muscles, and also improve the balance and coordination systems of your brain. As previously discussed, this balance and exercise input will help improve the function of all areas of your brain. Involving children with these exercises may help their neurological development and potential as well! In my office I use balance balls and other coordination and cerebellar exercises as part of the rehabilitation of children and adults that have behavior and learning problems such as ADD, AD/HD, OCD (obsessive-compulsive disorder), ODD (oppositional defiant disorder), PDD (pervasive developmental disorder), GAD (general anxiety disorder), NLD (non-verbal learning disorder), Asperger's syndrome, Autism, Tourette's syndrome, bipolar disorder, Dyslexia, Dyspraxia, and depression[9].

I teach exercise ball programs to my patients from a book titled *Therapeutic Exercises Using the Swiss Ball* (1994)[10], written by Caroline Corning Creager, P.T. In Ms. Creager's book, she illustrates over 250 different ball exercises. Some exercises are done in the sitting position (Fig. 14-1) and beginners should start here. Other exercises are performed in the supine position (Fig. 14-2), the prone position (Fig. 14-3), and in the bridge position (Fig. 14-4). I recommend her book for anyone interested in using a balance ball.

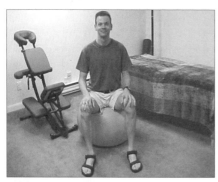
Fig. 14-1   Swiss ball - sitting

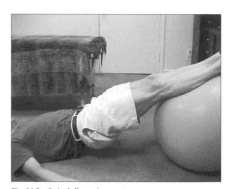
Fig. 14-2   Swiss ball - supine

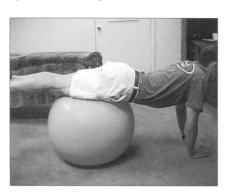
Fig. 14-3   Swiss ball - prone

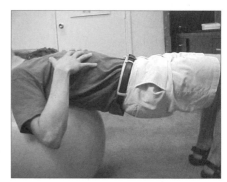
Fig. 14-4   Swiss ball - bridge

Swiss (balance) balls benefit the spine and nervou
ing flexibility, which helps improve the function of disc
When using balance balls, the receptors (nerve endings)
muscles stimulate nerve pools in the cerebellum and
proved health of nerve cells. By increasing the length a
on the balance ball, you can receive added cardiovasc
are exercise programs that exist with entire workouts o_
caution when performing abdominal exercises on the ball, especially those of
you with back pain (Chapter 8). Some of you may find abdominal exercises
on the balance ball helpful, but in my experience many people increase lower
back problems when doing abdominal work on the ball. Stick with the safe,
effective ab exercises discussed in Chapter 8.

ADDITIONAL EXERCISES

The next several exercises should be cleared by your doctor or therapist before
you begin. People respond differently to different exercises. I suggest trying
a variety of exercises, both the ones mentioned in this book and others you
may learn from other sources, and develop your own routine centered on the
exercises you respond to best.

Alternating Knee to Chest

Lie on your back either on the floor or on your bed with your knees bent (Fig.
14-5). Pull your right knee up to your chest as far as comfortably possible and
hold for a second or two (Fig. 14-6). Let that leg down and then pull the left
knee up to your chest (Fig. 14-7). Perform this exercise ten times per side and
be sure to keep both knees bent at all times. This exercise improves motion and
flexibility of the joints and discs of your lower back and helps stretch gluteal
and hamstring muscles. In this position, you can also perform a very gentle
but effective hamstring stretch by straightening and holding one leg at a time,
but keeping the knee slightly bent (Fig. 14-8).

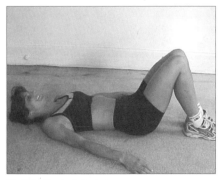

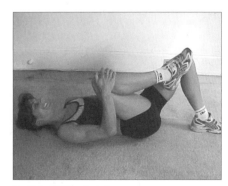

Fig. 14-5   Knee to chest - start

Fig. 14-6   Right knee to chest

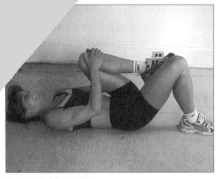

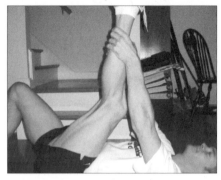

Fig. 14-7   Left knee to chest

Fig. 14-8   Easy hamstring stretch

Pelvic Push

This exercise will strengthen postural muscles of your middle and lower back and strengthen gluteal and hamstring muscles. Lie on your back with your knees bent and feet flat (Fig. 14-9). Raise your pelvis off the floor by pushing with your feet until your spine, pelvis and thighs are in a straight line (Fig. 14-10). If you are just beginning, try to hold this position for only a second or two. As you become more strong and stable, try to hold this position longer (5-10 seconds). Repeat as many times as comfortable and perform this exercise a few times a day in the beginning, gradually increasing the frequency over time. As always, reduce the intensity or stop the exercise if you feel pain. Some of you with low back pain will find this exercise comforting, while others will find it uncomfortable. If it is uncomfortable, obviously this is not an exercise to keep in your program.

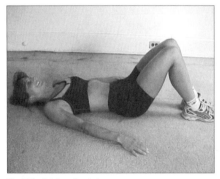

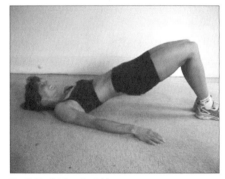

Fig. 14-9   Pelvic push - start

Fig. 14-10   Pelvic push - finish

Prone Extension

This exercise will assist in curve restoration and posture correction, and may help some of you with spinal pain syndromes, particularly neck pain, head-aches, and muscle tension and soreness in the neck, traps, and upper back.

Perform this exercise lying on your stomach. Your bed is probably the most comfortable place to perform this exercise, but you may also lie on carpet or an exercise mat. Place your arms alongside your body (Fig. 14-11) or bend your arms comfortably alongside your head (Fig. 14-12). Lift your chin first as if you are trying to look straight ahead (Fig. 14-13), then lift only your shoulders up a couple of inches (Fig. 14-14). Don't lift your shoulders any further than demonstrated here to avoid hyperextension of the lower back (Fig. 14-15). Hold the prone extension position for a couple of seconds at first and increase to ten seconds or more as you become stronger. Consider performing 2-3 prone extensions in the morning and again at night and increase as you see fit. The prone extension exercise, as with any other exercise, should be started slowly and decreased in intensity or stopped if you feel pain, discomfort or any other adverse symptoms.

The majority of patients I have evaluated have an increased curve of the low back, called *hyperlordosis*. In these cases, hyperextension of the lower back as shown in Fig. 14-15 may be damaging instead of helpful. The prone extension exercise may also be painful and usually avoided when someone has a

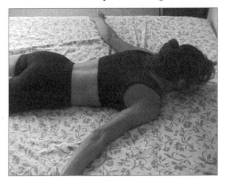

Fig. 14-11   *Prone extension - arms out*

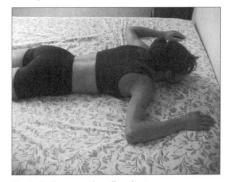

Fig. 14-12   *Prone extension - elbows bent*

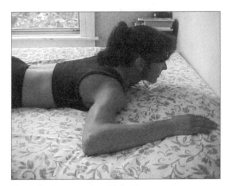

Fig. 14-13   *Prone extension - lift the chin*

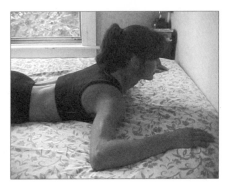

Fig. 14-14   *Prone extension, lift the shoulders gently*

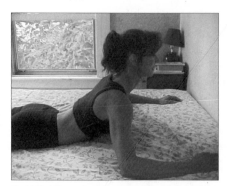

Fig. 14-15 This stretch may be a problem for some of you

spondylolisthesis, where one of the lumbar bones is erroneously positioned <u>in front of</u> adjacent bones. In contrast, some of you have a reduced lumbar curve (*hypolordosis*) and other conditions such as a *retrolisthesis*, where one of the lumbar bones is erroneously positioned <u>behind</u> the adjacent bones. People with hypolordosis and retrolisthesis may benefit from controlled hyperextension exercises as shown in Fig. 14-15. Hyperextension exercises should be performed under the advice and monitored by your chiropractor, therapist, or physician. Many of you reading this book are already performing hyperextension exercises taught to you by your therapist and have had positive results from doing so. Continue with your trainer's recommendation, especially if you have experienced measurable results and if the exercises are sensible for your condition. You can add this prone extension exercise I described here to your regimen, if and only if you receive measurable benefit.

Standing Distraction

I have a congenital condition in my spine called *facet tropism*. Facet tropism is when two joints of the same level of your spine are positioned in antagonistic alignment to one another, instead of being aligned in the same plane. Like most people, I am prone to having aches in my lower back if I am not careful with my day-to-day postures, positions, and ergonomics as described in this book. I am mindful about prolonged sitting, standing in one position, bending and lifting, and activities such as housecleaning. If I overexert myself, for instance helping someone move, I may have some low back pain at the end of the day, even though I am exceptionally careful to use my leg muscles to lift and not to bend at the waist.

In addition to utilizing good ergonomic habits and performing the flexibility exercises, I and many other people benefit from *distraction*. Distraction is where the joints of the spine are gently stretched apart. Distraction can be performed in many positions. Chiropractors and therapists, including myself, tend to perform distraction treatment in their offices with specialized tables and equipment. The equipment varies, and may position patients in the *prone* position (lying face down), the *supine* position (lying face up) or on an inversion unit that holds you upside down (Fig. 14-16). Flat, cot-like home distraction units are becoming popular (but please take your time trying a unit before you purchase one). Some of my patients respond well when I perform the *inversion* type of distraction shown in Fig. 14-16. Some of you with problems such as spondylolisthesis, retrolisthesis, hyperlordosis, disc syndromes, or facet tropism, may benefit from distraction in the office and at home. Again, you should only perform maneuvers like this under the advice of your health care practitioner. The way I like to perform distraction at home is by utilizing a countertop, especially a corner countertop. I place my hands flat on a countertop for support (Fig. 14-17). Keeping my arms stiff and very close to my body, I transfer my body weight onto my arms and hands and off my feet (Fig. 14-18). When performing this maneuver, the weight of the pelvis and legs will pull down, while the arms are pushing the weight of the upper body straight up, creating the distraction. This position can be held for several seconds if comfortable. As always, remember to keep your chin up. Depending on your height you may have to search for the appropriate height countertop or other strong fixed structure.

Some of you may benefit from simply hanging from your hands, perhaps in a gymnasium that has a high fixed bar (Fig. 14-19). This stretch does not work as well for my condition, but patients of mine have reported benefits from this type of distraction. Please start this maneuver slowly if you have never tried it before, and stop if it hurts. Other people I know have the older style gravity boots where you hang from a bar, but this method is considerably more difficult for most people to perform as compared to the methods described here.

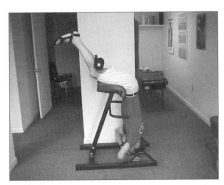

Fig. 14-16 *Inversion*

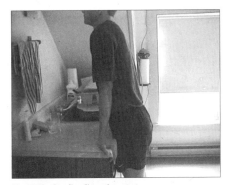

Fig. 14-17 *Standing distraction - start*

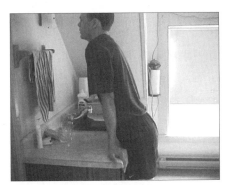

Fig. 14-18 *Standing distraction - finish*

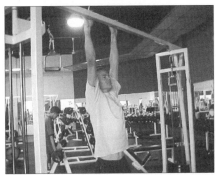

Fig. 14-19 *Hanging distraction*

Additional Ideas and Therapies

People with spinal pain have enjoyed improvements with other exercise programs and treatments such as massage therapy, acupuncture, martial arts, pilates, yoga, weightlifting, aerobics, dancing, and various physical therapy regimens. For example, my mother Joan who is 70 years young has battled low back pain and other various joint pains for decades. Regular wellness chiropractic care over 30 years has helped her enjoy a better quality of life. Recently she began participating in programs at the local YMCA, which include classes in aerobics, strength training, flexibility and yoga. Because she has certain limitations from her joint injuries, she modifies the workouts according to her ability, and follows the advice of the instructors. She attends the YMCA four days per week, totaling six hours a week of workouts. Of course, this is in addition to her ongoing daily spinal stretches (Chapter 2), walking, and gardening. Since starting these YMCA classes, Joan has enjoyed improvements in long-standing hip pain, flexibility, lower back pain, energy, focus, and restful sleep. The classroom exercises and stretches provided her with additional strategies to deal with her pain flare-ups at home.

In addition to specific food intake changes (Chapter 16) and increasing water intake, the exercise classes have assisted Joan in additional weight loss. In fact, extended family members mentioned during a recent gathering that she looks fabulous! Joan also likes to point out the social benefits of classes. She enjoys the interaction with other participants, as they laugh and support each other throughout the workouts. The social benefits result in improved attendance at the classes and follow-through with exercises at home.

15

BREATHING EXERCISES

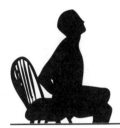

eep breathing is an important exercise that offers a variety of benefits. Many exercise programs including meditation, yoga, martial arts and some gym programs incorporate breathing exercises. Breathing exercises promote better movement of the rib cage, which increases joint and tissue nerve traffic to the brain. Breathing exercises also increase lung efficiency, improve oxygen levels in the blood, and help pump lymph fluid. More oxygen in the blood results in a healthier body, since oxygen is used in all bodily functions. The diaphragm has connections to the lumbar spine, so some people may notice improvements with low back pain from deep breathing exercises. Deep breathing exercises are easy and quick, and provide excellent benefits. You may want to teach breathing exercises to children to form an important early habit.

When you start breathing exercises, do them in a safe environment because of the potential of lightheadedness and dizziness. Sitting (and not driving) is the best way to begin. Start with one or two deep breathing exercises, because if you do too many you may become light-headed or dizzy or, in extreme cases, lose consciousness.

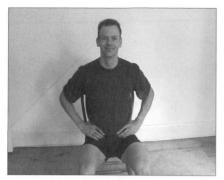

Fig. 15-1 Breathing exercise - start

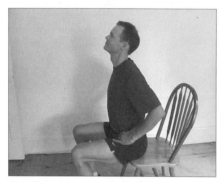

Fig. 15-2 Breathing exercise - shoulders back

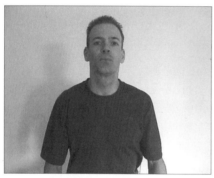

Fig. 15-3 Breathing exercise - exhale

1. Sit up straight with your head and eyes directed slightly upward (Fig. 15-1). This is to improve your posture and open up your rib cage.

2. Pull your shoulders back and place your hands either on your thighs, side, or in your lower back area, and slightly accentuate the curve of your lower back (Fig. 15-2). This will allow full movement of the ribs and diaphragm and help with lung expansion.

3. Begin by exhaling fully. Slowly take a deep breath in through your nose. Keep inhaling until your lungs are full, taking 4-6 seconds to do so.

4. Hold your breath for 3-10 seconds, but exhale immediately if you feel dizzy or faint.

5. Slowly exhale through your mouth with pursed lips to slow your exhalation (Fig. 15-3). Your exhalation time should be exactly <u>twice</u> your inhalation time. For example, if it took you four seconds to breathe in through your nose, take eight seconds to breathe out through your mouth. If you take five seconds to breathe in, take ten seconds to breathe out. The 2:1 ratio of exhalation to inhalation will take a little practice. Achieving this ratio trains your respiratory and nervous systems to maintain the proper 2:1 exhalation to inhalation ratio.

6. Maintain correct posture and repeat inhaling through the nose and out through the mouth.

7. Start slowly with only a couple of breaths per day. As you improve, work up to four deep breaths in a row, four times per day.

8. You can occasionally practice "abdominal breathing," which will target diaphragm motion. During one of your deep breaths in a four breath set, focus on "pushing your stomach out" during inspiration. With this focus you will notice your abdomen will fill more than your ribcage.

If you have difficulty with the breathing exercises when you begin, or if it has been a long time since you have exercised at all, start slow and be patient. Difficulty in the beginning illustrates the need for you to continue and improve. For those of you having difficulty at first, take an extended rest between deep breaths. You have plenty of time to improve. When you begin, it is helpful to have a partner count your inhalation and exhalation time. By using the partner method, you can also teach others to perform this very important and healthy exercise. Chiropractic treatment targets rib and spine flexibility, so consider a chiropractic evaluation if you think you have flexibility problems.

Arthritis is NOT a normal consequence of aging, and is mostly NOT caused by heredity.

> *"What do you expect? You're getting older, and you will have some arthritis."*
>
> *"Mom and dad had arthritis, that's why I do," is what many people are told and believe.*

This is not the case. Most arthritis is preventable, and many people suffering with arthritis pain can gain relief with a few lifestyle changes. Read on.

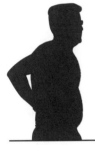

16

ARTHRITIS

T here are some important misconceptions about arthritis that I would like to address. I will offer references for those interested in investigating this subject further. The most important factor regarding arthritis is prevention. However, if you have arthritis, following the same advice for preventing arthritis can also provide great relief.

Misconception #1: Arthritis is due to old age.

This is simply not true. I have seen spinal arthritis on x-rays in 20-year old people and spinal arthritis-free people in their sixties and seventies. If arthritis was age-related, all joints would be equally affected. However, most people with arthritis have only one or several joints involved, not all joints. I have observed many cases of arthritis affecting certain areas of the body in some people and other areas in other people. Certain individuals have more systemic inflammatory arthritis that I will discuss later.

Misconception #2: Arthritis is a consequence of injury.

This is only a partial truth. A joint that is injured may experience accelerated wear and tear (*osteoarthritis*) as compared to uninjured joints. You will learn that wear-and-tear arthritis is not only due to injury and usage, but diet.

Also, injured joints that are "arthritic" and painful can benefit greatly from improved dietary habits.

Misconception #3: There is no known cure for arthritis.

I disagree, as do many other physicians, researchers, and former arthritis pain sufferers. The majority of arthritis is due to poor diet, therefore if someone is suffering from swollen, painful, angulated, worn joints and they change their food selection dramatically, the pain and swelling of the arthritis may diminish. Again, the most important aspect of arthritis is prevention. If you prevent it, you never need to treat it, or find a "cure." If you do have arthritis, dramatic food selection changes may provide significant symptom relief.

Misconception #4: Arthritis runs in families.

Not at all. The majority of arthritis is not due to bad genes or faulty heredity. It is mainly due to poor food choices, that were passed down from mom and dad (and society) to the children. This misconception that arthritis runs in families has been formulated by simple observations. When parents have arthritis and then their children have arthritis, the easy but erroneous conclusion is that it was passed down from parents to children, and it "runs in the family." However, observing arthritis in two generations does not prove that faulty genes are passed down; certainly bad habits are passed down. We tend to have the same nutritional habits as our parents, therefore we tend to get similar diseases, including arthritis (or heart disease, or cancer, or diabetes, or obesity, or osteoporosis). There are other factors that result in a population with poor eating habits. The food delivery system in the US provides too many products that taste great, are cheap, and readily available ("fast food"), but are really, really bad for us. These processed foods are laden with refined carbohydrates and sugar, and too much protein (especially animal protein). They also contain bad fats (saturated, hydrogenated, and trans-fats), and often have added taste enhancers, called excitotoxins, similar to MSG. I will discuss these issues in another book.

There are several types of inflammatory arthritic disorders, including rheumatoid arthritis (RA), systemic lupus erythematosus (SLE, or lupus), gout or gouty arthritis, psoriatic arthritis and ankylosing spondylitis (AS). Many medical professionals and groups, including the Arthritis Foundation, have stated that food has nothing to do with arthritis. However, there is almost no medical literature to substantiate this viewpoint. Growing amounts of research demonstrate a strong relationship between diet and arthritis. My experience continues to fortify this link between certain foods and arthritis.

Gout or gouty arthritis ("rich man's disease") is caused by a diet high in purines. Foods that are high in protein from animal sources are the foods that are rich in purines. Purines are broken down in the liver into uric acid.

Increased animal protein intake results in an increase in purines and this in turn causes an increase in uric acid production. Uric acid crystals deposit in joints, making them painful and swollen. Attacks of gout tend to begin suddenly and also tend to go away with or without medication. Almost all doctors now agree that gout has a dietary link and medical research supports this. A simple solution to prevent gout (or to improve an existing gout condition) is to decrease or eliminate foods high in animal protein (beef, chicken, fish, dairy, eggs, etc.). If you suffer with gout, and you decrease animal protein, you may not notice complete relief of pain. Complete elimination of animal foods may be necessary to totally relieve your pain. This goal of complete elimination presents obvious problems, since many people are unwilling to totally abstain from animal foods. One of the toughest problems I have encountered in clinical practice is getting people with arthritis (and other conditions) to eliminate animal protein from their diet. Those that do enjoy massive benefits and significant or total resolution of their pain.

Osteoarthritis is the most common type of arthritis and is generally considered to be age-dependent and due to wear and tear of joints. However, osteoarthritis is not an inevitable result of age. It is true that activities which result in injuries can lead to higher levels of osteoarthritis. Sports such as football, hockey, boxing, basketball, volleyball and running, among others, may lead to accelerated joint problems, but other steps can be taken to minimize the amount of osteoarthritis. The food you eat is the most important factor determining how much arthritis you will have, and how much you will hurt from it.

More on age and arthritis.

Osteoarthritis is not a normal consequence of aging. It has been observed that osteoarthritis is rare in certain parts of the world. For example, people in Africa are essentially free of osteoarthritis even though they perform hard physical labor until late in their lives. You will learn that one of the main factors which determine how much arthritis you get is the food you choose to eat.

The microcirculation (capillaries) which supplies blood to the joints is compromised by a high saturated/hydrogenated/trans-fat, high cholesterol, high calorie, and high processed food American diet. This adversely affects the health of the joints and obstructs healing. For many of you, changing to a lower protein, healthy fat, whole grain (low glycemic index), no processed food, and high-plant based diet will give your body the best chance to heal bone and joint surfaces and tissues, reduce systemic inflammation, and reduce pain. If you suffer from joint pain, you may benefit from purified fish oil supplements (see reference pages), which should only be taken under the advice of a qualified health care professional, especially if you are taking blood-thinning drugs. I have seen wonderful improvements in patients with arthritic pain when they take fish oil and antioxidant supplements. Fish oil is powerfully anti-inflammatory, which helps fight inflammation and pain.

Several types of arthritis are grouped together as inflammatory arthritis, including rheumatoid, gout, lupus, psoriatic arthritis and ankylosing spondylitis. These types of arthritis are rare in regions of the world where animal products are seldom eaten and diets are starch, vegetable, and fruit-based, such as Africa and Asia. These inflammatory diseases are caused when the immune system makes antibodies to fight what the body determines as foreign substances (antigens). Often the antigen (the bad guy) is protein, and for many people, it is animal protein. This results in antigen-antibody complexes, which lodge in various tissues, causing inflammation and pain. Once again, the high bad fat, high animal protein, highly processed American diet will compromise oxygen delivery to joint tissues, resulting in further antigen-antibody complexes to form in the joints. After eating a single meal that is high in fat and cholesterol, blood thickening (sludging) occurs, which reduces oxygen transfer into joints, leading to more inflammation. Even some plant fats such as vegetable oils can add to blood sludging and joint inflammation and pain, especially when combined with animal and processed foods.

Lupus is less common in Chinese people who live in China as compared to Chinese people who have moved to Hawaii and adopted the typical American diet, loaded with animal foods rich in antigenic proteins, bad fats, cholesterol, antibiotics, growth hormones, and pesticides. Ankylosing spondylitis is an arthritic condition that mainly affects the spine and hips. This disease is much less common in countries with a starch or plant-based diet as opposed to countries with a high bad fat, animal-based diet such as in the United States. Psoriatic arthritis sufferers may also benefit from more of a plant-based diet as described.

According to information in Dr. John McDougall's book, McDougall's Medicine[11], dairy foods are the most common source of the antigens involved with inflammatory arthritis, with eggs being a close second. Beef is another common antigen-producing food. Some people are allergic to plant foods, such as wheat and corn, causing joint inflammation. For people who suffer with arthritic pain, eliminating dairy, eggs and beef (and possibly chicken and shellfish) may result in dramatic improvements in their pain, suffering and inflammation in a very short period of time. Some people need to eliminate all animal protein to gain the pain relief their bodies are screaming for. There are ways to find out which foods are aggravating your pain. One way is called an elimination diet (described in Dr. McDougall's book and in other sources). Another way is to receive a very specific blood test to identify food allergies (not environmental allergies such as pollen, dust, and animals). Blood allergy testing[12] should be conducted by a health care practitioner familiar with this type of testing. If you have inflammatory arthritis or osteoarthritis, consider having a blood food sensitivity test to help identify which foods are causing inflammation and pain. The exact foods which aggravate inflammation will differ, sometimes greatly, from person to person. For more information regarding blood food allergy testing, see the reference page.

If you decide to get a blood food sensitivity test, follow the instructions of the lab and your doctor carefully. Results you are hoping for with the dietary changes may not be immediate. After the "elimination" phase, you can put the results to the test. If you decide to reintroduce the offending foods, you may notice pain and inflammation return. If so, you have all the evidence you need.

Dr. McDougall also states that drugs should be reserved only for those cases that fail to respond to changes in diet. Many of the drugs prescribed for arthritis have serious side effects and complications, which need to be considered. Typically there are no negative side effects with healthy dietary change, and often other health problems (heart disease, most cancers, diabetes, obesity, digestive disorders and osteoporosis) may greatly improve with changes in diet.

Please note that I am not stating that you must become a strict vegetarian to see your pain diminish, or to prevent arthritis. Some of you may have to, but some of you may need a blood test to determine your specific sensitivities, and some of you may need multiple strategies such as fish oil, antioxidants, chiropractic care, and other treatments for best results.

In Dr. Andrew Weil's book, Eating Well for Optimum Health[13], he recommends eliminating vegetable oils, margarine, shortening, all partially hydrogenated oils, and all deep-fried foods to help improve arthritis. He recommends using extra-virgin olive oil as your main fat, increasing your omega-3 fats, and eating more fruits and vegetables. Dr. Weil also believes you can possibly reduce or get off arthritis drugs with diet changes as discussed. The typical Western diet promotes inflammation, and by adjusting the fats you eat and eating more anti-inflammatory foods, you may be able to reduce drug dosages. In my opinion, Dr. Weil's book is one of the best books written about nutrition and health.

A research article titled "Controlled Trial of Fasting and One-Year Vegetarian Diet in Rheumatoid Arthritis" was printed in the British journal called "The Lancet" in October, 1991. In this research, the control group ate an ordinary diet, while the experimental group fasted for 7-10 days, then new foods were introduced. If a new food caused joint pain and swelling, it was eliminated for the following year. At the end of one year, the physical condition of the people in the control group (eating an ordinary diet) deteriorated. The experimental group, which ate an individually adjusted vegetarian diet, enjoyed reductions in joint pain, stiffness, and swelling, among other indicators.

Joint pain increases when the inflammation levels in those joints increase. If you have a chronic pain syndrome, including spinal pain, you should consider a significant change in food as a primary strategy on regaining your health and reducing your pain. Remember that significant dietary change should be made under the advice and consultation of your healthcare professional. Reducing animal foods is a good idea as these foods are high in cholesterol, saturated fat, calories, and have no fiber. In addition, extra weight that you carry causes added pressure and irritation to the discs and joints of your spine. This is an additional contributor to spinal wear and tear and chronic pain syndromes. Shifting to more of a plant-based diet can help safely remove unwanted, damaging pounds in a healthy manner, allowing you to once again enjoy your work, home, relationships, play time and hobbies.

Many of us tend to choose the easiest solution to a problem. This is particularly true for many Americans regarding their health. Many people choose low personal effort when dealing with their health issues, and these treatments often include drugs and surgery. However, medical research is clear: The vast majority of degenerative conditions are highly preventable and treatable through improved lifestyle, mainly diet and exercise. However, this involves higher personal effort. My personal experience with thousands of patients has shown that only a small number of people are willing to make significant food changes, even though these changes may result in wonderful reductions in pain and improvements in health.

Removing processed food, soda, and other beverages may also help improve your pain. Processed foods (anything with a package) often have taste enhancers, processed carbohydrates, high fructose corn syrup, and other additives that can increase pain. Consider significant reductions or elimination of processed foods, soda, and juice for yourself and your children. Water should be your preferred beverage. Read "Excitotoxins: The Taste That Kills" by Russell Blaylock[16]. This book will enlighten you about chemicals added to food that are potentially damaging and dangerous.

For references and additional reading materials, please see the back of the book.

In conclusion, if you have arthritis and arthritic pain, or want to avoid arthritis and arthritic pain, here are several helpful options.

1. Eat more vegetables and non-citrus fruit

2. Eliminate dairy products

3. Eliminate all processed, packaged food, including soda and "sport drinks"

4. Take fish oil and antioxidant supplements (under your doctor's supervision)

5. Consume less animal protein, and some of you may need to eliminate all of it

6. Get a blood food sensitivity test to accurately determine which foods to eliminate

7. If you don't get a blood test, and if you are very disciplined, consider an elimination diet or fast, and then add foods one at a time to determine which ones cause pain.

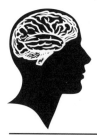

TECHNO BABBLE

I n this last chapter I would like to provide some of the scientific research that explains how chiropractic treatment affects the nervous system, how chiropractic can help those in pain, and help people stay healthy and well. The exercises, stretches, and ergonomic changes discussed in this book may not be enough to alleviate the pain that some people have. In my opinion the strategies in this book are most effective at keeping you healthy and well when used in conjunction with ongoing chiropractic care. I frequently tell patients it is easier to keep someone well who is already well than try to fix someone who is broken.

This thought can be applied to the entire health (disease?) care system in this country. Many of the most profound and memorable results that I and other chiropractors have observed have not only been with pain cases but with other types of health issues such as ear infections, asthma, migraines, ADD, AD/HD (and other learning and behavior issues) and, in the early days of chiropractic, flu and polio. I am not stating that chiropractic was a cure for these problems; rather, chiropractic care promoted changes in the nervous system, which led to improvements in the health and function of other systems in the body.

I will keep the explanations brief and as easy as possible to understand. This chapter will be more technical, so it may not be suited for everyone. Read on to learn about the effects of chiropractic care on the nervous system, spine, and pain.

The nervous system controls all body functions and activities. The condition of your nervous system ultimately affects the health and performance of your body, which determines your ability to enjoy relationships, work, play time and hobbies.

NUTRITION AND BRAIN HEALTH

The basic building block of the brain and nervous system is the neuron—the nerve cell. A neuron requires several things in order to live and function properly: the macronutrient glucose (and other macronutrients, as Dr. Andrew Weil states) and micronutrients. Glucose is fuel of cells and is derived mainly from the dietary intake of carbohydrates, and to a smaller extent, fats and proteins. Fats and proteins are also needed in appropriate amounts and types to have healthy cell structure and repair, and for production of neurotransmitters, hormones, and enzymes.

My food recommendations are similar to the Japanese way of eating, as most Japanese are thin, enjoy low disease rates and have excellent longevity. I recommend a diet focused on lots of fresh vegetables and fruit, low glycemic index starchy carbohydrates (beans, rice-except short grain white rice-yams, sweet potatoes), some cold water fish (non-farmed, non-atlantic wild salmon, mackerel, herring, sardines, anchovies), and whole, stone-ground grains and bread.

I believe that complete elimination of dairy products is a good idea, particularly for infants and children, as it is a common allergen, high in contaminants, and may be the cause of a variety of other health problems and chronic pain. More on that in subsequent books. I also recommend a significant reduction or elimination of meat and poultry, which contain a variety of health hazards including inflammatory-inducing proteins that cause chronic pain.

Cold water fish supplies nerve cells with vital Omega-3 fats EPA (Eicosapentaenoic acid) and DHA (Docosahexaenoic acid). The brain is comprised of 60% fat, much of which should be EPA and DHA. Many people, particularly in America, are very deficient in EPA and DHA, and eat too much saturated fat, hydrogenated fat, and trans-fats from processed and animal foods. These bad fats decrease the performance of the nervous system and also contribute to the strength of pain pathways.

I also recommend purified fish oil supplements (see reference pages) for a number of my patients, but check with your health care professional who is knowledgeable about them before taking any. Decreasing saturated, hydrogenated, and trans-fat intake may help protect people from other health problems such as heart disease, cancer, arthritis, and obesity.

I also strongly recommend the complete elimination of all processed foods especially for infants and children. These foods are laden with processed carbohydrates (white flour and sugar), hydrogenated and trans-fats, and *excitotoxins*[16]. Excitotoxins are food additives similar to MSG, which are hidden in food as glutamate, "natural flavors," hydrolyzed soy and vegetable protein, and sometimes soy protein isolate. Please note if foods contain these items in their ingredients, it is not a guarantee that excitotoxins exist. Some "natural flavors" may indeed be natural. I recommend you contact individual manufacturers to accurately identify suspect ingredients before eating them or giving them to your children. Processed foods and additives adversely affect nerve cell health, enhance the pain pathways, and lead to obesity.

THE IMPORTANCE OF OXYGEN

Neurons also need oxygen and there are many factors involved in oxygen absorption and delivery. One is rib cage motion and flexibility. The deep breathing exercises described in Chapter 15 are helpful in maintaining full rib cage excursion. Appropriate thoracic (middle back) and lumbar (low back) biomechanics, posture and flexibility are important to respiration as well. This is an additional reason why proper posture as described throughout this book is so important, and a reason why regular chiropractic (wellness) care benefits your health. Rib cage function can be improved with exercises, chiropractic care and awareness of how to use your body during the day. The diaphragm is a flexible dome-shaped membrane and is the essential muscle of inspiration. It has attachments to the ribs and lumbar spine, therefore compromised lumbar spine and rib cage flexibility and posture may interfere with diaphragm activity and the ability to take in oxygen.

Blood vessel diameter is controlled by the *sympathetic nervous system* (SNS). It is critical for a healthy functioning body that sympathetic activity is controlled appropriately. The cortex (brain) regulates sympathetic activity, therefore cortical health has a large influence on the SNS. With proper brain health, the output of the SNS is properly regulated, allowing certain blood vessels to remain at larger diameters, which allows better oxygen and fuel delivery to neurons and other cells. Brain health is largely determined by what you eat, how much you exercise, the health and condition of your spine (chiropractic, spinal exercises, posture), and how you use your body during each day.

THE BRAIN'S POWER SOURCE

Another critical item that nerve cells need for survival and health is called *activation*. Activation means that a nerve cell is being electrochemically stimulated to work via neurotransmitters released by other neurons that act upon it. Appropriate activation stimulates the neuron's internal mechanisms which keeps it alive. These mechanisms include energy and protein production, neurotransmitter manufacture, and DNA and RNA replication, which lead to healthier cell membranes, efficient ion pumps, and stronger cell structure. Essentially all internal cellular activities improve with appropriate activation. If activation of a cell drops enough and for a long enough period of time, the neuron's health will decrease and it may die, and certain neurons cannot be replaced.

As a simple example to demonstrate activation, consider how you feel after you exercise. You tend to be more awake and better able to concentrate. If you are in decent cardiovascular fitness and work out regularly you tend to be more awake, feel more alive and perhaps even be happier. If you have had a spell of inactivity you tend to be fatigued, stressed and less productive. While exercising, you stimulate nerve receptors in your joints and muscles which activate neurons in your brain. Another reason to exercise regularly! This is similar to increasing the power to a light bulb; it will shine brighter and reach its full potential.

What you eat plays a large role in activation too. Excitotoxins and trans-fatty acids in processed food and a lot of fast food alter neurotransmitter levels, creating an unhealthy environment for neurons. They fire too much and become exhausted. For example, some people don't feel well after consuming MSG (monosodium glutamate), which is an excitotoxin. Low consumption of fruits, vegetables, and whole grains decreases antioxidant intake, which decreases neurons' ability to dispose of metabolic waste and free radicals properly; thus, nerve cell toxins accumulate.

EXERCISE YOUR BRAIN

The types of activities that are important for brain health are clear. Dr. Dan Murphy brought a couple of research articles to my attention in July 2000, which describe the activities that improve the health of neurons. The first article, "The Brain is Like a Muscle,"[17] describes that neurons need to be stimulated to stay alive and to function properly. The report showed that cognitive activity such as learning a new language, solving puzzles and performing hobbies keep neurons active and healthy. Physical activity drives receptor systems that have similar effects on the brain. Of course, exercise has multi-faceted, positive impacts on the body including improved musculoskeletal health, cardiovascular benefits and keeping nerve cells healthy via increased activation. The article indicates that some brain diseases such as Alzheimer's disease and dementia could be prevented with cognitive exercises and physical activity. Dietary factors were also discussed in this article. The second article[18] described how consumption of vegetables seems to have healthy benefits to neuron health and survivability. Eating more vegetables and grains help keep blood vessels clear and provide nourishing essential fatty acids and antioxidants for the brain as previously mentioned.

CHIROPRACTIC EFFECTS ON THE BRAIN AND ON PAIN

Chiropractic care was not mentioned in these articles but the effects of chiropractic care offers similar neurophysiological benefits. Chiropractic spinal manipulation and other chiropractic methods including specialized table treatments and instruments are commonly called adjustments. These adjustments stimulate special nerve sensors called receptors, which are buried in many of the tissues of the body. The most important receptors that have the greatest impact on brain health are those receptors that are sensitive to motion and gravity. These receptors are called mechanoreceptors and muscle spindles, and are located in joint tissues, ligaments, skin, muscles and tendons. The highest concentrations of these receptors are found in the joints, discs, ligaments and muscles of the spine, especially the cervical spine. Chiropractic adjustments specifically target these tissues and their receptors, which offer the greatest activation of the brain. The positive effects of chiropractic adjustments may last long after the treatment is over. Chiropractic treatments may reduce joint and tissue malfunction and scar tissue, improve motion of spinal joints, discs, and tissues, and improve our relationship with gravity. These joint dysfunctions are commonly referred to as spinal *subluxations*. Reduction of these joint dysfunctions or subluxations may lead to richer mechanoreceptor and muscle spindle activity to the cerebellum and cortex. These receptors powerfully stimulate nerve cells in the brain.

To sum up this technical description, my colleague Dr. Dan Murphy explains the effects of chiropractic adjustments this way: "Chiropractic adjustments use the bones of the spine as levers to stimulate joint mechanoreceptors and muscle spindles, in an effort to abort the neurological maintenance of pain and disease."[19]

Science now tells us that the *cerebellum* (in the back portion of the head) actually operates first in both cognitive and motor activities. This means that the cerebellum plays an important role in a variety of cortex activities (probably all), not just motor activities as previously thought. Therefore, the development, health and function of the cerebellum will ultimately affect the development, health and function of the cortex.

Neurons of the cerebellum are primarily driven by the activity of muscle spindles throughout the body. Joint mechanoreceptors stimulate the cortex mainly via the thalamus, and are also extremely important for the health of the brain. The highest concentration of joint mechanoreceptors and muscle spindles are found in the tissues in an around the spine as mentioned. Therefore, the health and activity of each joint, disc, ligament, and muscle of the spine is critical for appropriate activation of nerve cells in the cerebellum and cortex. Chiropractors specialize in identifying dysfunctional motor units of the spine and extremities and chiropractic treatment is focused on improving the function of dysfunctional joints. Chiropractic adjustments both stimulate mechanoreceptors and muscle spindles, and are focused on improving joint,

disc, and muscle dysfunctions. Adjustments may have a brief effect by stimulating these receptors, but more importantly a lasting benefit by reducing the
joint dysfunctions for sustained firing of these receptors long after the treatment. The adjustments also improve our relationship with gravity, creating
additional lasting stimulation of the brain. All of the receptor stimulation will
improve the critical activation of nerve cells of the spinal cord, cerebellum and
cortex. The firing of mechanoreceptors and muscle spindles also helps fight
pain by stimulating the release of pain-inhibitory neurotransmitters, which is
why many people enjoy pain relief with chiropractic treatments. The adjustments may benefit people in pain a secondary way, by improving the health
of the stuck, glued, painful joint(s), which is often the original source of pain.
Please note that singular joint problems of the spinal discs and joints often cannot be exercised or stretched out, meaning that stretching and exercising cannot be a complete replacement for chiropractic adjustments. Improved posture
and ergonomic habits, stretching, and general physical exercise described in
this book should be used in conjunction with chiropractic care, not as a replacement.

TECHNO BABBLE SUMMARY

As a review, the amount of muscle spindle and joint mechanoreceptor activity
on an ongoing basis plays an extremely important role in the development
and health maintenance of the of the human brain. This realization has been
the basis of chiropractic treatment since 1895, even though we have not known
how chiropractic influenced the nervous system until the middle to latter part
of the twentieth century. As knowledge of the function of the nervous system
grew, we could better understand and explain the results that patients enjoy
after receiving adjustments from a chiropractor. In my opinion, and I think
many would agree with me, chiropractic is not the only way to stimulate these
pathways. However, chiropractic care delivers a unique stimulation to the human nervous system that no other treatment modalities can provide. When
people have spinal intersegmental joint dysfunctions (subluxations), exercise
alone cannot correct the problem. Since chiropractic taps into the network of
receptors which are highly concentrated in and around the spinal tissues, chiropractic plays and will continue to play an increasingly important role in
healthcare. Of course, many joint dysfunctions and subluxations can lead to
inflammation and pain, which is why many people seek out chiropractic care
for spine and extremity pain, and why many people enjoy relief of pain from
chiropractic adjustments. Many chiropractors, like myself, advocate coming
in for maintenance and wellness chiropractic treatment, before joint and disc
dysfunctions become painful and arthritic, and before they significantly impact nerve cell health. Also, maintenance and wellness chiropractic treatments
are more cost effective, because the visits tend to be much lower in frequency
as compared to crisis, pain relief care.

Spinal stresses lead to wear and tear, loss of motion, and poor relationship with gravity, ultimately decreasing the activity of the cerebellum and cortex. Improving spinal function and stimulation of the brain has been the purpose of this book. Many of our day-to-day activities accumulate stress within the spine and decrease spinal flexibility, and may lead to joint dysfunctions (subluxations). A decrease in spinal function will then decrease receptor activation of neurons in the cerebellum and cortex. This decrease could lead to a variety of problems and symptoms that people experience. Decreasing the amount of spinal stress that we endure during each day, performing the exercises described in this book, and being checked on a periodic basis by a chiropractor will help increase the stimulation of receptors to activate the neurons of the cerebellum and cortex. Improving spinal health as described in these ways will fight pain and ultimately improve function of all systems in your body.

General physical exercise performed throughout your life should be an absolute top priority for anyone that has the ability to perform exercise. The physical activities chosen will vary from person to person but they all have a common denominator. When you move joints and muscles, receptor activity increases, which will activate the cells of the spinal cord, cerebellum, and cortex, improving overall health. Exercise, coupled with posture awareness, ergonomic improvements, improved nutrition, and chiropractic check-ups may also help to avoid childhood (ADD, AD/HD, etc.) and adult (Alzheimer's disease, dementia, Parkinson's disease, etc.) brain dysfunctions. With my patients, I consistently use a simple example of garbage in, garbage out. Good stuff in, good stuff out. This means if you improve the muscle spindle and mechanoreceptor activity to the brain, you will improve the output of the brain (in general). Living a sedentary lifestyle has several ill effects on health, one of which is decreased stimulation and function of your nervous system.

The recommendations I make to patients regarding ongoing chiropractic treatment may be different than those of other chiropractic practitioners. This disparity from one doctor to the next is similar to other healthcare professions, meaning the recommendations given by practitioners in a certain field will differ from one to the next. I recommend that people seeking treatment from a chiropractor or another healthcare practitioner should simply feel comfortable and understand the treatment program that their practitioner offers. In my office I have a goal to see patients as infrequently as possible once their major problems, dysfunctions, and subluxations have been dealt with to keep their nervous system functioning appropriately. But, I recommend a lifetime of care and maintenance for families, especially babies and children. This is quite different than developing a treatment strategy based on pain and disease only. Chiropractors in general tend to be proactive regarding health, meaning we try to convey ideas to our patients on how to stay healthy and well, rather than waiting for disease and breakdown to occur in the body. One of the analogies I use is similar to automobile maintenance. We all know it is important to have regular oil changes even though the car appears to be running well. My recommendations to my patients are much more important than an oil change, and I make these recommendations to try to keep people healthy instead of waiting for the engine to blow, and then trying to "find a cure" for the blown engine. In essence, I consistently promote "health" care, rather than "disease" care.

Many people seek care from chiropractors and other healthcare practitioners for relief of pain. Pain is important and passionate for many and those that suffer with pain find that their work, relationships, play time and hobbies are adversely affected. In all of the tissues in your body you have pain nerve endings called *nociceptors*. When tissues become irritated, nociceptors are stimulated and send pain information to the brain. If enough nociceptor (pain) nerve endings are stimulated, the person will have a perception of pain. Pain can also be increased by other factors as well. Poor dietary habits will change the internal chemistry of your body, and promote higher concentrations of inflammatory substances that stimulate nociceptors, increasing pain. Decreased functioning of the cerebellum and cortex may lead to an increased perception of pain. The muscle spindles in muscles and mechanoreceptors in joints, ligaments, and discs coexist with nociceptors. This means that when tissue is less flexible, injured, scarred, or irritated, the mechanoreceptor and muscle spindle traffic decreases. Nociceptor traffic replaces the mechanoreceptor and muscle spindle traffic, which may lead to the perception of pain. Think of hot water and cold water out of a faucet. If you have appropriate amounts of hot and cold water, the water feels comfortable and warm. If the cold water (mechanoreceptors, muscle spindles) is turned down or shut off, you are left with hot, scalding, painful water (nociceptors). A wonderful way to improve this situation is to increase the flow of cold water to result in comfortable, warm water. Even if the hot water (pain) is decreased in flow, the water that is coming out of the faucet remains hot and painful. The analogy is similar to relieving pain pathways with painkillers only, which might not be the best long-term strategy for somebody suffering with pain. One excellent way to decrease and possibly eliminate pain is to increase the flow of cold water, meaning to increase the activity of mechanoreceptor and muscle spindle activity, while addressing the source of pain, which may be joint dysfunctions, subluxations, scar tissue, and inflammation.

Hopefully the information transmitted in this book will be shared and many may benefit. Improving the ways that you use your body during the day with concentration on ergonomics, performing simple daily spinal exercises, improvements in diet, decreasing stress and evaluation by a chiropractor are all excellent strategies to help you maintain a better level of health. If your health improves you have an increased ability to enjoy your work, relationships, playtime, sports and hobbies. Please feel free to contact me with feedback regarding the activities that I described in this book. This will help me develop more helpful tools in the future so we all have a chance to enjoy better health and a Happy Back.

INFORMATION PAGES

FIND A DOCTOR OF CHIROPRACTIC IN YOUR AREA

If you do not already have a chiropractor, word of mouth is a great way to find one. Talk to your family, friends, and co-workers, and find out whom they recommend. Often you can visit a chiropractor for a consultation or some sort of an introductory health class to get a feel for the doctor or clinic before undergoing treatment. If you do not find any referrals this way, try the organizations below.

Chiropractic Biophysics (CBP) Practitioners:
Use the Chiropractic Biophysics webpage, www.idealspine.com, click on "find a chiropractor."

Massachusetts Chiropractors:
www.MassChiro.org, click on "Find a Doctor."
This site has additional health information and research.

Chiropractic Pediatrics and research in Chiropractic for pregnancy and children:
Try the website for the International Chiropractic Pediatric Association, www.icpa4kids.com, click on "Find a Doctor of Chiropractic."
This site has additional information on how to have healthier babies, children, and families.

For additional information, and to find other Doctors of Chiropractic across the nation and in other countries, contact the International Chiropractors Association, www.chiropractic.org.

You can also try the American Chiropractic Association for more information and to find a chiropractor:
www.amerchiro.org.

FISH OIL AND SUPPLEMENTS

I recommend liquid instead of gelcaps. Liquid fish oil is usually substantially cheaper when you compare milligrams of EPA and DHA per serving. EPA and DHA are the important fats in fish oil, and their concentration in milligrams will be listed on the label. You will need gelcaps for travel, as bottles of fish oil need to be kept refrigerated when opened, whereas gelcaps are stable at room temperature for periods of time. I recommend taking antioxidant supplements, specifically coenzyme Q-10, alpha-lipoic acid, Glutathione, B and C vitamins, magnesium, and selenium, along with fish oil. The Nutri-West supplement company (below) has a supplement that has all of these products in one tablet.

Only use fish oil products that mention "purified with molecular distillation," "pharmaceutical grade," and/or "no detectable levels of mercury, PCB's, or other heavy metals and contaminants" on their label. These products will cost a little more, but in my opinion it is critical and worth the extra cost.

Carlson Labs:
www.carlsonlabs.com. Try "The Very Finest Fish Oil," or "Cod Liver Oil" for winter months in colder climates (lack of sun and vitamin D).

Nutri-West:
www.nutri-west.com. Try "Complete High-Potency Omega-3 Liquid," and "Complete Omega-3 Co-Factors." They also have products for pregnant and lactating women, babies, and children. Products from Nutri-West are only available through doctor's offices.

Nordic Naturals:
www.nordicnaturals.com. They have omega oils for pets, too.

FITNESS AND WELLNESS INFORMATION

www.heartzones.com
Sally Edwards is a talented athlete, educator, author, and speaker. She is the founder and CEO of Heart Zones, a training and education company. This website is full of information to help you improve and monitor your health and fitness. This website is for fitness beginners up to competitive athletes and professionals.

Carmichael Training Systems: www.trainright.com.
Chris Carmichael was one of Lance Armstrong's coaches. His website and company is loaded with training advice for all sports and all levels of fitness and competition.

www.mercola.com
Dr. Joseph Mercola has one of the most popular health and wellness web sites on the internet. His site has an easy search area which accesses thousands of pages of easy to use advice to help you get and stay well. For additional information on chiropractic, type "chiropractic" in the search box.

www.highandtightfitness.com
Bill Murphy is a certified personal trainer, certified diet and nutrition specialist, certified Fitness Coordinator, WNBF Professional Bodybuilder, and a published author. He is in the Woburn, Massachusetts area.

NUTRITION INFORMATION AND ADDITIONAL READING

The Crazy Makers-How the Food Industry is Destroying Our Brains and Harming Our Children. By Carol Simontacchi. Tarcher/Putnam, NY, 2001. A fantastic book which I highly recommend.

Eating Well for Optimum Health, by Dr. Andrew Weil, MD. Knopf, NY, 2000. Dr. Weil has a tremendous amount of information available through his books and website, www.drweil.com.

The McDougall Program for Women, by Dr. John McDougall, MD. Plume, NY, 2000. Dr. McDougall also has a tremendous amount of information available at www.drmcdougall.com.

Everyday Cooking with Dr. Dean Ornish, by Dr. Dean Ornish, MD. HarperCollins, NY, 1996. Dr. Ornish has more information at www.ornish.com.

Diet For A New America, John Robbins, HJ Kramer, Inc., 1987. EarthSave International, PO Box 96, New York, NY, 10108, (800) 362-3648, www.earthsave.org.

For additional information about a pain-free back and a healthy lifestyle: *Taking Your Back to the Future*, by Dr. Michael Gazdar, DC. John Muir Chiropractic Center, Walnut Creek, CA, 1995.

Terry Marotta is an experienced non-fiction writer, a syndicated columnist and four-time author. See more about her work at www.terrymarotta.com.

Model: Ann Coros
Ann is a gifted athlete and model. Her information can be viewed at: www.trislp.com.

REFERENCES

1. Kellett, John. "Acute soft tissue injuries-a review of the literature." *Medicine and Science of Sports and Exercise, American College of Sports Medicine* 18 (5; 1986): 489-500.

2. *Sports Medicine: Prevention, Evaluation, Management, and Rehabilitation*, Steven Roy, M.D., and Richard Irvin, Prentice-Hall, Inc., 1983.

3. Dr. Dan Murphy, personal communication and class notes.

4. Drawing by Faith Brosnan, April 2006. Adapted from *The Physiology of the Joints*, Kapandji, I.A., Churchill Livingstone, 1974.

5. Adapted from Wikipedia.org. www.wikipedia.org/wiki/Image:Gray_111_-_Vertebral_Column.png. Originally from *Gray's Anatomy*.

6. Nachemson, AL. "Disc Pressure Measurements." Spine 6 (1; Jan.-Feb. 1981): 93-7.

7. Wilke, HJ, et. al. "New in vivo measurements of pressures in the intervertebral disc in daily life." Spine 24 (8; 1999): 755-762.

8. *Taking Your Back to the Future*, Dr. Michael Gazdar, John Muir Chiropractic Center, 1995.

9. *Neurobehavioral Disorders of Childhood*, Robert Melillo and Gerry Leisman, Kluwer Academic/Plenum Publishers, 2004.

10. *Therapeutic Exercises Using the Swiss Ball*, Caroline Corning Creager, Executive Physical Therapy, Inc., 1994.

11. *McDougall's Medicine*, John A. McDougall, M.D., New Win Publishing, Inc., 1985.

12. Sage Systems, Inc. laboratory, www.foodallergytest.com, 800-491-9511; Cell Science Systems, www.alcat.com, 800-881-2685; Immuno Laboratories, www.immunolabs.com, 800-231-9197; Great Smokies Diagnostic Laboratory, www.gdx.net, 800-522-4762.

13. *Eating Well for Optimum Health*, Andrew Weil, M. D., Alfred A. Knopf, 2000. www.drweil.com.

14. *The Crazy Makers; How the Food Industry is Destroying Our Brains and Harming Our Children*, Carol Simontacchi, Tarcher/Putnam, 2000.

15. *Diet for a New America*, John Robbins, HJ Kramer, Inc., 1987.

16. *Excitotoxins: The Taste That Kills*, Russell Blaylock, Health Press, 1997.

17. Neergaard, Lauran. *"Scientists Urge Mental Exercise."* Washington, AP, 7-24-00.

18. Pennell, Mary. *"Vegetables High in Antioxidants May Reduce Risk of Alzheimer's Disease."* Washington, Reuters Health, 7-17-00.

19. Dr. Dan Murphy, class notes, 1991.

INDEX

Activation, 103
ADD (Attention Deficit Disorder), 84, 107
AD/HD (Attention Deficit/Hyperactivity Disorder), 84, 107
Adjustments (chiropractic), 18, 60, 105
Airbags, 30
Allergy Testing, 98
Alzheimer's Disease, 107
Antigens, 98
Arthritis
 ankylosing spondylitis (AS), 96, 98-99
 arthritis foundation, 96
 and diet, 96-99
 and genetics, 96
 gout, 96-98
 lupus (SLE), 96, 98-99
 and old age, 95
 osteoarthritis, 1, 2, 95, 97-98
 psoriatic, 96, 98-99
 rheumatoid (RA), 96, 98
Asperger's Syndrome, 84
Atrophy, 16
Autism, 84
Avascular, 16

Benign Paroxysmal Positional Vertigo (BPPV), 74
Biking
 aero position, 69
 hybrid, 69
 mountain, 69
 postures, 69-71
 recumbent, 77-79
 upright, 77-79
Bipolar Disorder, 84
Bone Spur, 16

Cancer, 96, 99, 102
Car Seat Position, 30

For more information and healthy advice, please visit Dr. Fuller's website:

www.drscottfuller.com

DR. SCOTT FULLER, D.C., C.C.S.T., D.A.C.N.B.
Doctor of Chiropractic
Chiropractic Certification in Spinal Trauma
Diplomate of the American Chiropractic Neurology Board

Dr. Scott E. Fuller, D.C., C.C.S.T., D.A.C.N.B., is a 1984 graduate of Peabody High School (Peabody, MA). He received an Associate in Arts/Pre-Chiropractic degree from North Shore Community College in 1986 (Beverly, MA) and his Doctorate of Chiropractic Degree from Palmer College of Chiropractic in Davenport, IA in 1989. He has been in clinical practice ever since. Dr. Fuller has devoted much of his post-graduate effort to research as well as clinical experience. He received his C.C.S.T. (Chiropractic Certification in Spinal Trauma) in 1996, and a 3-year, 360-hour postgraduate neurology D.A.C.N.B. degree (Diplomate of the American Chiropractic Neurology Board) in 2002. Dr. Fuller is also a noted teacher and lecturer, and conducts presentations on a variety of healthcare subject matters at schools, companies, organizations, and in his private chiropractic practice.

He maintains a private chiropractic practice (Fuller Chiropractic, P.C.) in Woburn, MA, since 1993. Dr. Fuller received a Competent Toastmaster designation (CTM) from Toastmasters International in 1997. Dr. Fuller currently lectures on ADD, AD/HD (and other learning and behavior disorders), brain nutrition, disease prevention, stress management, exercise and improving sports performance, chiropractic, ergonomics, motivation, work safety, and other health and wellness subjects. Dr. Fuller also has a local cable television show in the Woburn area entitled "Health Source," which he began in 1996. Health Source has aired for the past 12 years with over 200 episodes completed. Fuller Chiropractic publishes newsletters for patients and interested parties regarding important health issues on an ongoing basis, much of which can be found on his website, www.drscottfuller.com.

Dr. Fuller continues to be a competitive athlete. He was a runner in junior high and high school. He was a bodybuilder in graduate school, and was the training partner of a competitive bodybuilder. After playing volleyball in the mid-90's, he has been competing in triathlons since 1999, encompassing various distances, including 2 ironman triathlons and 2 stand-alone marathons. He has competed in several bike races since 2001. Currently he competes in shorter distance events, including sprint triathlons, bike races, and running events.

CONTACT INFORMATION

You can contact Dr. Fuller the following ways.

Office:
Dr. Scott Fuller
Fuller Chiropractic
576 Main St.
Woburn, MA 01801
781.933.3332

Website:
www.drscottfuller.com

E-mail:
drscottfuller@aol.com

HAPPY BACK
Order Form

Number of copies: _____ @ $15.95 ea.   = $_____

Shipping: $2.95 per book   = $_____

                                  Total   = $_____

Please send check or money order with the bottom half of this page to:

Fuller Chiropractic
576 Main St.
Woburn, MA 01801

Please indicate the address where you want to receive your books.

For credit card orders, please call 781-933-3332.

For more information and healthy advice, please visit Dr. Fuller's website:

www.drscottfuller.com

CONTACT INFORMATION

You can contact Dr. Fuller the following ways.

Office:
Dr. Scott Fuller
Fuller Chiropractic
576 Main St.
Woburn, MA 01801
781.933.3332

Website:
www.drscottfuller.com

E-mail:
drscottfuller@aol.com

HAPPY BACK
Order Form

Number of copies: _____ @ $15.95 ea.   = $_____

Shipping: $2.95 per book   = $_____

                                            Total   = $_____

Please send check or money order with the bottom half of this page to:

Fuller Chiropractic
576 Main St.
Woburn, MA 01801

Please indicate the address where you want to receive your books.

For credit card orders, please call 781-933-3332.